Infection Control

How to Implement an Effective Approach for Long-Term Care

Brian Garavaglia, PhD

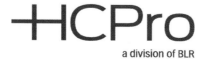

a division of BLR

Brian Garavaglia, PhD, Author
Olivia MacDonald, Editor
Erin Callahan, Vice President, Product Development & Content Strategy
Elizabeth Petersen, Executive Vice President, Healthcare
Matt Sharpe, Production Supervisor
Vincent Skyers, Design Services Director
Vicki McMahan, Sr. Graphic Designer
Sheryl Boutin, Layout/Graphic Design
Reggie Cunningham, Cover Designer

Advice given is general. Readers should consult professional counsel for specific legal, ethical, or clinical questions.

Arrangements can be made for quantity discounts. For more information, contact:

HCPro
100 Winners Circle, Suite 300
Brentwood, TN 37027
Telephone: 800-650-6787 or 781-639-1872
Fax: 800-785-9212
Email: *customerservice@hcpro.com*

Visit HCPro online at *www.hcpro.com* and *www.hcmarketplace.com*.

Contents

Chapter 1

Purposes and Objectives

Introduction

The necessity for a sound infection control program in long-term care cannot be understated. In fact, in any area of healthcare, infection control is of paramount importance. This is well documented by the sheer number of nosocomial (health facility acquired) infections and iatrogenic (conveyed to patients through healthcare provider contact) infections each year. Infection control practices must be understood to varying levels by all healthcare professionals, regardless of whether one is an administrator, director of nursing, physical therapist, physician, or dietician. Only through a well-implemented comprehensive infection control program can healthcare facilities effectively limit the spread of infections among patients and workers.

This book can be a template for all healthcare organizations; however, it is specifically focused toward the long-term care environment. While a bacterial or viral agent does not change from one healthcare environment to another, certain infectious agents may be more commonly found in certain environments based on the specificity of clientele that they serve. This book will examine the nature of infection control as it is specifically related to the long-term care environment.

Effective infection control programs need all individuals in the healthcare facility to have varying levels of education and knowledge to forestall the transmission of infectious agents that can become epidemic in the healthcare facility. Certain individuals, such as the infection control nurse or medical director, are expected to have greater levels of knowledge regarding infection control. However, an effective infection control program must pervade all aspects of the environment in order to enhance the health and wellbeing of all residents and workers alike.

The objectives discussed in this chapter will guide the development and evaluation of an infection control program and drive the coordination of activities so that the reader will be able to employ a coordinated and systematic endeavor to successfully implement an infection control protocol with an organizational mindset. This chapter will lay the foundation for the rest of the book. It will start with explaining why infection control is so critical for long-term care. It will also acquaint the reader with what a sound infection control program provides to the long-term care environment.

The Purposes of an Infection Control Program

Think of the purposes of an infection control program as its intended results—what does it attempt to accomplish? Here are some purposes to consider for your program.

Control the transmission of infection among the long-term care staff, its residents, and the residents' families

To accomplish this, an infection control program needs to:

- Create policies and procedures that address infection control issues
- Ensure that the care for each patient consistently incorporates appropriate and correct infection control practices
- Educate staff, residents, and family members on relevant infection control issues and practices
- Monitor infection control trends
- Take action to improve care delivery in light of infection control principles

Ensure compliance with regulations

The *Conditions of Participation* expect the healthcare organization to maintain an effective infection control program as part of its overall quality assessment and performance improvement efforts. Surveyors scrutinize care delivery practices during the survey process, and an increasingly important area of concern is infection control.

Government agencies such as the Occupational Safety and Health Administration (OSHA) and the Centers for Disease Control and Prevention require the agency to enforce the use of stringent hand washing techniques, follow universal precautions and infection control principles, and implement exposure control programs.

Finally, healthcare organizations must also comply with local laws regarding the reporting of communicable diseases to local health departments, as well as follow these local organizations' guidelines for properly handling and disposing of contaminated materials and infectious waste.

Given the large array of federal, state, and community level organizations that often demand compliance on infection control issues such as monitoring and reporting of communicable illnesses, the Centers for Medicare and Medicaid Services (CMS) have amalgamated all of these agency concerns on infection control, including their own, and developed an overriding regulatory requirement. This regulation is often referred to as F-tag 441. It reads as follows:

F-tag 441

F441 (Rev. 127, Issued: 11-26-14, Effective: 11-26-14, Implementation: 11-26-14)

§483.65 Infection Control

The facility must establish and maintain an Infection Control Program designed to provide a safe, sanitary and comfortable environment and to help prevent the development and transmission of disease and infection.

§483.65(a) Infection Control Program

The facility must establish an Infection Control Program under which it:

    (1)   Investigates, controls, and prevents infections in the facility;

    (2)   Decides what procedures, such as isolation, should be applied to an individual resident; and

    (3)   Maintains a record of incidents and corrective actions related to infections.

§483.65(b) Preventing Spread of Infection

    (1)   When the Infection Control Program determines that a resident needs isolation to prevent the spread of infection, the facility must isolate the resident.

    (2)   The facility must prohibit employees with a communicable disease or infected skin lesions from direct contact with residents or their food, if direct contact will transmit the disease.

    (3   The facility must require staff to wash their hands after each direct resident contact for which hand washing is indicated by accepted professional practice.

§483.65(c) Linens

Personnel must handle, store, process and transport linens so as to prevent the spread of infection.

The above regulation was taken from CMS' State Operations Manual. F-tag 441 deals with the promulgation of regulatory requirements dealing with infection control. Infection control has taken on a greater importance in long-term care due to the increasing numbers of often preventable hospitalizations related to infections. Also, the ever-increasing level of antimicrobial resistance has been a driving force in heightened regulatory surveillance given by surveyors to infection control issues in long-term care. Moreover, the need to provide a safe and healthy long-term care environment that minimizes the communicable transmission of disease-causing pathogens to residents, workers, and visitors is the goal of this important regulation.

Long-term care environments deal with those who are sick and often quite infirm. Minimizing the transfer of often preventable infectious agents has become an increasing priority. Eliminating unneeded hospitalizations due to preventable infections helps to minimize runaway costs that are found in our healthcare system, and controlling the transmission of pathogenic agents to already sick and frail individuals can prevent these individuals from needlessly becoming more ill or even dying. Finally, a strong infection control program saves money for the healthcare facility on the operational level and provides for a more functional resident population, as well as a healthier workforce.

The rationale for starting this book with CMS' regulatory requirement for infection control is that a clear delineation of this regulation will be the framework for the rest of the book. Since the regulation has become increasingly paramount in the minds of surveyors, it also needs to be paramount in the minds of those who work within the long-term care environment. This book is specifically aligned to address the importance of the infection control requirement with the hope of helping to prevent long-term care facilities from receiving the often-cited F-tag 441 for noncompliance in this area.

Ensure compliance with state and federal regulatory standards as well as accrediting organizations

For long-term care, especially nursing home regulatory compliance, state and federal requirements are of foremost importance. However, since many healthcare facilities, including long-term care facilities, are seeking additional accreditation with organizations such as The Joint Commission, infection control standards are closely scrutinized. Even OSHA, with its fairly recent focus on long-term care facilities, has taken an interest in infection control, bloodborne pathogens, and proper protection for workers in these organizations. One of the most important needs within a long-term care organization is an infection control program that implements and coordinates policies and procedures to lower the risk of infection among staff, patients, and family members, and to improve the trends and rates of infections. An effective infection control program includes:

- Infection control policies and procedures to provide education, surveillance, identification, reporting, prevention, and control of infections
- Uniform compliance guidelines for universal blood and body fluid precautions and consistent monitoring procedures
- Ways to evaluate the efficiency of their infection control programs

Ensure timely response and appropriate actions in cases of resident infections and exposure incidents

The agency must have methods to identify and track infections and exposure incidents, as well as mechanisms to improve performance and reduce adverse events. These should be part of your quality assurance program, which along with the infection control committee, should make sure that proper tracking methods are being implemented assiduously and correctly. More will be said about monitoring and tracking later in this book.

Validate that agency policies and procedures incorporate infection control principles

Each of an agency's policies and procedures must reflect sound infection control theory and practice. The agency must establish a method to develop, implement, review, and revise policies and procedures. Moreover, these policies must not be formulated in a cursory manner, but must be based on appropriate empirical support and scientific evidence. It is important that the policies and procedures that are implemented are efficacious as demonstrated by scientific support for their use and implementation.

Ensure that documentation in clinical records, incident reports, and staff health records is accurate and demonstrates appropriate services and actions

The long-term care facility must maintain records supporting their actions and interventions. Documentation must accurately reflect compliance with regulations and standards and demonstrate that the healthcare facility provides appropriate services, that meet appropriate standards to maintain the health and safety residents and workers.

Ensure that the agency's quality improvement processes incorporate and address infection control issues

In order to succeed, a long-term healthcare facility's quality assessment and improvement program and committee (QA) must integrate all important infection control processes, such as tracking the types of infections occurring each month, possible location of the infection's source, reports on any cultured organisms that may pose more than an ordinary risk to the long-term care community, as well as records for preventative interventions, such as vaccinations for residents and workers alike. These are just a few of the things that need to be targeted by an infection control committee as part of the QA process.

The Objectives of an Infection Control Program

Clear objectives drive an infection control program. Remember, objectives are different from goals in that they are more specific and explain how you will carry out your program. You need to make sure your objectives are not only clear, but realistic. In order to satisfy regulatory and accreditation requirements and keep your staff and residents safe from infection, you should strive to meet the following objectives in your infection control policy.

Describe the scope and requirements of the infection control program

- List those staff who are required to participate in the infection control program
- Make sure each staff member's requirements and responsibilities are specifically outlined
- Define areas of responsibility and accountability for education, monitoring, and follow-up
- Include discussion on staff and patient communicable diseases
- List all the procedures that staff must practice throughout care delivery

Implement a comprehensive staff education program

- Outline the kinds of material you will teach staff, residents, and residents' families regarding infection control practices
- Educate staff on every aspect of your infection control program, including identifying parameters for ongoing education
- Establish guidelines for resident education on infection control techniques in the home

Establish a clear sequence of events in the surveillance, identification, reporting, prevention, and control of infection to ensure appropriate services and timely action

> **Surveillance, identification, and prevention** are probably the most important factors for infection control. In an era when we have an increasing number of pathogens that are no longer responsive to many antibiotics available, the best way to treat infections and infectious potentialities is to eliminate them before they happen or attack them during their incipient stages.

- Define all of your infection control procedures (e.g., hand washing, universal precautions, nursing bags, personal protective equipment, etc.) intended to reduce the spread of infection among staff, residents, and residents' family members
- Devise a reporting mechanism when new infections and exposure incidents are suspected
- Identify the source and extent of the problem, as it possibly could exist if nothing is done
- Specify procedures for monitoring the status of known infections (in both staff and resident populations) and medical follow-up for exposure incidents
- Develop the exposure control plan—review and update it annually to ensure all staff are trained accordingly
- Create guidelines for hepatitis B vaccinations and TB skin testing
- Implement a respiratory protection plan
- Track and report all infections
- Evaluate your research, and plan and implement a control strategy

Demonstrate compliance with local, state, and federal laws, requirements, and accreditation standards

- Check all federal and state regulations and accreditation standards, identify their intent, and recognize how to demonstrate compliance in everyday care delivery practices
- Establish guidelines for the infection control practices, handling, and disposal of infectious waste to comply with these requirements (e.g., proper disposal of biohazard elements such as waste and needles)

Provide methods for accurate documentation in clinical records, incident reports, and staff health records

- Define the frequency for clinical record review related to infection control practice and surveillance
- Specifically define who will be responsible for these reviews—especially in addition to the medical director and director of nursing
- Establish how staff are to document their adherence to infection control policies
- Review incident report forms and infection logs to ensure accuracy
- Maintain confidentiality of staff medical information, and make sure it is in separate files from other personnel information
- Inform and remind staff of the absolute necessity for complete documentation and follow-up of all observations

Establish guidelines for staff interaction with residents, families, caregivers, and coworkers that promote appropriate surveillance, prevention, and control of infection

- Set risk assessment guidelines to evaluate the healthcare environments after discharge for resource availability problems (e.g., no running water in the home, pest infiltration, etc.) and knowledge deficits of family caregivers (e.g., the only caregivers who may not have a sound understanding of assisting the resident after discharge with such things as wound care utilizing an aseptic field)
- Create guidelines for identifying resident and family education issues

Ensure adequate data collection, analysis, assessment, and interpretation of infection findings

- Maintain adequate data collection regarding infection information, staff exposure, and trends within your resident census
- Identify the specific resident populations and procedures with higher probabilities of infection or exposure risk
- Commit quality resources to analyze infection trends and initiate action plans if infection rates in the agency exceed acceptable limits

Develop specific objectives and outcome measures to assess the effectiveness of the infection control program

- Formulate an infection control committee to carry out the objectives of the program, assess whether the program is meeting its goals, and evaluate the program quarterly (but preferably monthly) for any needed changes or updates
- Integrate the committee activities with the healthcare facility's quality assessment and process improvement program (QAPI)

INFECTION CONTROL PROGRAM
Purpose(s): The purpose of [facility name]'s infection control program is to guide our employees in the prevention of and/or limit the exposure to infectious diseases and/or infections.
Objectives:
1. Decrease risk of exposure to infections 2. Decrease risk of exposure to infectious diseases 3. Reinforce staff knowledge of infection precautions/prevention 4. 5. 6.
Signature   Date
Signature   Date

Although this book attempts to provide considerable coverage of infection control, it is by no means an exhaustive compendium of the topic. However, the goal is to provide long-term care staff with a better knowledge of infection control. It is not just targeted at a small group of individuals with select skills. Its goal is to help enhance the skills of all professionals within long-term care. Therefore, although some information may be more relevant for some professionals than others, the goal is to provide broad coverage of the many facets of infection control that can have some applicability for all long-term care professionals. In addition, it is the hope that those who read this book will find it relevant toward maintaining compliance with CMS' regulatory requirements in this area as well as helping to build a culture within long-term care that is increasingly knowledgeable about infection control and sensitive to its concerns.

Chapter 2

Principles of Disease

This chapter will focus on communicable diseases, which are transmittable from one person or organism to another. Infection control is highly interested in the communicability of microorganisms that can cause disease. Microbial agents, such as bacteria, viruses, fungi, parasitic agents, etc., play an important role in infectious disease, especially those that have higher levels of communicability or levels of virulence that can severely compromise the health and welfare of a healthcare facility's environment. It is important for those within healthcare facilities in general, and long-term care facilities in particular, to have some level of working knowledge about the principles of disease. For instance, many pathogenic agents that are part of any healthcare environment carry varying potential for causing disease. I am reminded here about the words of one of my microbiology professors regarding microbes. He stated that even when we are handling and culturing organisms that may not be highly virulent, we must not fall prey to mishandling and improper antiseptic procedure, since ALL microbes carry the potential for being pathogenic, and therefore, disease-causing. These are wise words to remember.

Important Disease Classifications

There are two principal terms that are often mentioned when one speaks about disease: acute versus chronic diseases. Acute diseases are relative severe, but they are characterized by a more sudden onset and shorter duration. Conversely, chronic diseases have a much longer and often continuous duration, and many have no cure.

Do not be fooled into thinking that acute diseases, because they are shorter in duration, are less severe. These two terms do not indicate severity. In fact, acute diseases such as cholera or Ebola can kill quickly. Also, take for instance the bite of a tick, which can lead to an acute rash and other minor symptoms, but can also cause Lyme's disease and have devastating and ravaging chronic effects on the health of a person that may leave them infirm and even cause death in the long-run.

Communicable diseases

Communicable diseases, which can be transferred from one person or organism to another, are contrasted with noncommunicable diseases, such as osteoarthritis or cardiovascular disease, which are not able to be transferred from one person to another. Communicability is based on the virulence, or the potency of the disease-causing pathogen (organisms or agents that cause disease). For instance, the human immunodeficiency virus (HIV) was, and still is, highly feared. However, its communicability is limited. It is typically only able to be transmitted through direct contact with body fluids. This is not to say that it is not highly virulent. However, its virulence is dominant once it has entered into the body of the person. Outside of the body, it is easily destroyed and has limited communicability.

We can also use the acute and chronic classification to examine these two diseases. The HIV virus is a communicable disease agent that when transmitted to another person, leaves the person with a chronic disease. The treatment emphasis is palliative, attempting to prevent further exacerbation toward the more lethal acquired immune deficiency syndrome (AIDS). Conversely, the influenza (or flu) virus strikes the person quickly, typically has a short duration of a week or less, and is highly communicable. The flu virus is more emblematic of an acute disease or illness. Influenza is often a seasonally-based communicable disease that has to be addressed regularly in long-term care environments. However, diseases such as HIV are also increasingly found within nursing home residents today because many individuals are living longer with the virus due to the following:

- improvement in pharmacological intervention
- younger individuals being found in nursing care settings, especially within post-acute care
- diminished fear of taking individuals into long-term care settings with such microbial diseases due to better education and training

Agent, host, vector, carrier, and vehicle

Other important public health concepts include the following terms: agent, host, vector, carrier, and vehicle.

Agent

An agent is the source or cause of a disease. Whether it is a poison ivy plant causing poison ivy dermatological manifestations, or a living organism, such as a bacterium infecting a person and causing tuberculosis, these are all infecting agents.

Host

A host is a living organism that harbors a disease, often without showing any symptoms of the disease. Using the example of HIV infection, those who are infected with the virus are hosts. Animals may be hosts for a number of diseases that can be passed on to humans through their milk products or through being eaten, leading to them becoming not only the host, but an agent for the transmission of the disease-causing organism and subsequently, the disease in itself.

Vector

Vector is sometimes used synonymously with agent in that it is often defined as any agent, such as a human being or animal, that transmits an infectious agent or organism into another organism. Vector has also been used more specifically to refer to invertebrate animals, especially arthropods such as mosquitoes, fleas, ticks, and mites that carry infectious agents. Mosquitoes carrying the bacterium for malaria, the rat flea that transmits bubonic plague, and the deer tick that transmits Lyme disease are some common arthropods that are vectors for these diseases.

Zoonosis is the transfer of a disease-causing agent from an animal to a human being. Where vector has been commonly used for infectious agents transferred by invertebrates, zoonoses are those diseases that are transferred from vertebrate organisms to humans. Rabies transferred by a rabid dog, a vertebrate, to a human through a bite would be an example of a zoonotic infection. Other forms of zoonoses include Creutzfeldt-Jakob disease from the cow or bubonic plague from infected rats.

An important concept that often is mentioned in discussing infection control by health professionals is the concept of the reservoir or environment in which the infectious agent lives, multiplies, and grows. As one can see, targeting the reservoir of microbial elements can be very important to slow down growth and replication and, ultimately, to stop the growth and development of an infectious agent. This could encompass a humidifying ventilation system, a refrigerator at an inappropriate temperature that encourages microbial growth or reproduction, a mold buildup that spreads infectious spores within an environment, or even a person, who is not only a reservoir, but also a host.

Carriers

Healthcare and infection control personnel have to be aware of the concept of carriers. A carrier is a person or animal that carries an infectious/pathogenic agent and, therefore, holds the potential to infect a large amount of the population with whom they may come into contact. For instance, many work areas, especially healthcare work areas, require tuberculosis testing and possible chest x rays to monitor for those who may have tuberculosis or be active carriers of the disease organism. Carriers, such as the well-known case of Typhoid Mary, can be insidious, since in many cases they may not present any outward disease manifestations or be sick themselves, yet they nevertheless can still transmit their pathogenic organism to others and make them ill.

Furthermore, visitors to a healthcare facility, including both people and pets, may act as carriers, bringing with them parasites and other microbial agents, that can quickly infect a population, and especially cause significant implications for those who may be immune-compromised.

Vehicles

Another term that is often used by those within the infection control area is vehicles for the transmission of disease. Vehicles are nonliving substances that contribute to the transmission of infectious agents. Often the technical term "fomite" is used to refer to an inanimate source that harbors infectious agents. For instance, a countertop may contain bacteria that contribute to disease. Reusable cloth towels that many housekeepers and staff use to clean multiple tables may also contain infectious agents that transmit disease-causing agents. Even a stethoscope used for frequent physical examinations without being sterilized can carry bacteria that may act as a vehicle, or fomite, that transmits pathogenic bacteria.

Common Modes of Disease Transmission

A few major modes of disease transmission that will be discussed here. These modes of transmission are central to understanding disease. It is paramount that long-term care professionals become acquainted with these major modes to properly address infection control in their facilities.

Direct transmission

Direct transmission refers to the direct contact between the infectious agent or host and the organism that the disease agent is transmitted to. Person A, who is infected with HIV, having unprotected sexual intercourse with person B and subsequently transferring the virus to person B is an example of direct transmission. In long-term care, a person with *Clostridium Difficile* (C. Diff) on their hands may come into contact with another resident and transmit the infectious agent. Or a resident, family member, or worker with conjunctivitis may transmit the infectious agent to another person directly through unwashed hands that they rubbed their eyes with.

Indirect transmission

Indirect transmission happens when there is an intermediate vehicle involved in the transmission of a disease-causing agent. For instance, if a person wiped his or her nose on a hand towel, then placed it back on the towel holder and someone else dried his or her hands with the same towel and became infected, the infection would have been indirectly transmitted. Merrill (2010) stated that various forms of indirect transmission can exist. One major form of indirect transmission is airborne transmission. Sneezing and coughing are common modes of airborne transmission. Moist, airborne particles, aerosolized in the air, disseminate through the immediate environment and are breathed in by those within that environment, infecting these individuals.

Vector-borne and vehicle-borne transmission can be found in infectious agents transmitted by arthropod organisms. Zoonotic agents can be included here as well. Other vehicle-borne agents, such as fomites, are instrumental in the transmission of disease. Inanimate objects such as, countertops, chairs, drinking glasses, drinking fountains, or curtains, may contain many disease-causing pathogens.

Disease Progression

One might ask the question, "Why do we have to discuss disease progression in regard to an infection control program?" Although disease progression can entail both acute and chronic illnesses, the concern for long-term care facilities is with the more acute and infectious agents that can cause disease. Furthermore, having some understanding of the progression of disease also helps you recognize the resources and urgency with which you must address a particular matter. Understanding the progression of a disease as it may possibly be passed from one person to another can determine how you act to address a specific case and prevent it from leading to epidemic proportions within your healthcare facility.

Merrill (2010) delineated the natural history of the disease process. If no medical intervention exists, there is a natural progression of steps that follow in the disease process with some level of predictability. The following is the delineation of the natural history of disease progression, emphasizing the communicable disease process. Although it is not the focus of this book, many forms of noncommunicable, chronic forms of disease could also be delineated through this process as well.

Stage one: Susceptibility

In this stage, there is no disease. It is the stage that precedes the disease itself; the disease is not evident in the person or the individual has not been introduced with an infectious agent that will cause the disease. However, the person's level of susceptibility is important at this point. Some individuals will be more susceptible to certain diseases. Moreover, at this stage, primary prevention can be very important in forestalling disease. Infectious disease committees in long-term care should be emphasizing this stage to prevent further disease from happening. Since many individuals in long-term care facilities have some level of compromised immunity, these individuals are prime candidates for many infectious agents to be introduced into the population and cause disease that would not be caused in more immune-healthy individuals. These opportunistic infections, infections that are not normally caused by microbes in otherwise healthy individuals, are preventable. Yet, one must understand their population, the level of acuity and susceptibility, and then work to address their infection control needs based on this level. For instance, as individuals reach older ages, the immune system becomes slightly more compromised, which may make those individuals more susceptible to disease. Also, at this point, having proper inoculations are an important form of prevention that can reduce disease susceptibility.

Stage two: Pre-symptomatic disease

During this stage, the person is now infected with the disease-causing agent or has disease progression taking place within the body. After exposure to a disease causing agent, there is often an incubation period where the disease is replicating, yet no symptoms are evident. This latency period is the period from the time of initial exposure that initiates the progression of a disease to the presentation of the actual symptoms of the disease (Merrill, 2010). During this stage, secondary prevention therapeutically attempts to prevent the disease or illness from progressing or even attempts to eliminate the disease altogether.

Stage three: Clinical disease

This is the stage that is most commonly associated with the disease process. It is the point in the natural history of disease progression in which symptom manifestation develops. Clinical signs and symptoms indicative of specific types of diseases are now apparent, and a diagnosis is usually forthcoming. If the disease previously existed at the subclinical level, it now is manifesting itself at the clinical level. Secondary prevention may continue to exist at this level to address amelioration of the disease. Tertiary prevention may also be instituted for addressing chronic issues that may need palliation. Many individuals at this stage of disease may also end up within an acute care setting, such as a hospital, for further treatment.

Stage four: Recovery, disability, and death

In this stage, the person, depending on the type of disease, the disease's virulence, the extent of the disease's insult to the body, and the quality of treatment available to the sick individual, not to mention the premorbid health status of the resident, will help to determine whether the individual will recover, remain disabled, or die. An elderly, frail individual with compromised immunity may die from the influenza microbe. However, other individuals with a greater resiliency may weather the acute infectious condition with no more than a couple of days of feeling poor.

Immunization in Long-Term Care

Immunization has been one of the greatest advances in helping people live longer and more disease-free lives. It has been one of the most important areas of primary prevention. Due to immunization, we have nearly eliminated many common scourges of the past, such as death from small pox, diphtheria, and polio. The Centers for Disease Control (CDC) view immunizations as possibly the greatest advance in enhancing our overall wellbeing, writing:

> Perhaps the greatest success story in public health is the reduction of infectious diseases resulting from the use of vaccines. Routine immunization has eradicated smallpox from the globe and led to the near elimination of wild polio virus. Vaccines have reduced some preventable infectious diseases to an all-time low, and now few people experience the devastating effects of measles, pertussis, and other illnesses. (CDC, "History of Vaccine Safety")

We often think of immunization being important for young children. However, individuals within long-term care facilities need to follow a successful immunization program led by the infection control team to ward off many forms of preventable illnesses. This is especially important beacuse many older adults are more susceptible due to reduced immune responses. Furthermore, proper documentation of records and specific vaccinations are often required for infection control, and it is an area that is carefully examined by survey officials that come in for annual facility inspections.

With the work of Edward Jenner successfully providing inoculation and protection against smallpox in the late eighteenth century, the importance of immunization was well on its way. Vaccine development proliferated. Louis Pasteur was instrumental in the development of vaccines to protect against anthrax and rabies. However, probably the most recent successful immunization effort was brought forth by the genius of Janus Salk, whose work on the polio vaccine led, a half century later, to our world virtually achieving his sought-after goal—the complete eradication of polio. These important public health measures are now important practices used to control the health of the long-term care environment. Furthermore, if implemented and monitored assiduously by an infection control team, the preventative benefits for maintaining a healthier long-term care environment are immeasurable.

Understanding immunity

Although long-term care personnel are not typically involved in the clinical realm of immunity and immunology other than through the administration of vaccinations, they still have to be conversant with the area of immunity. This is especially important today because immunization has become a preventive force within long-term care. Given this, having a working knowledge of some of the more important concepts of immunity is necessary for all healthcare professionals to be able to converse with other professionals on this important health issue, whether working within a community or an acute or long-term care facility. In examining immunity, the first differentiation that has to be made and known about is between innate and acquired or adaptive forms of immunity.

Innate immunity

Innate immunity is present from the time of birth. These are often numerous nonspecific factors that exist during times of disease. Physical barriers, such as the skin and mucous membranes, chemical or naturally produced enzymatic agents, fever, inflammatory responses, and phagocytic activity, make up the innate system.

Acquired or adaptive immunity

Acquired or adaptive forms of immunity are achieved through the natural process of the body's immune system coming in contact with microbial agents that stimulate the immune system, subsequently producing antibodies against the naturally occurring microbial agents that the individual encountered through their daily interactions with their environment. This is typically referred to as a naturally occurring acquired immunity, since they acquired the immunity without any type of artificial assistance. Furthermore, when a person acquires an illness and produces antibodies during that illness from their B-lymphocyte production, this is also considered part of the naturally acquired immunity. This often happens to many who work in healthcare. They find themselves often getting sick upon entering a new facility, being exposed to microbes that are endemic to the healthcare environment. They eventually come to develop a naturally acquired form of immunity to the endemic infectious agents in the environment.

Acquired or adaptive immunity can also be achieved through an artificial mode. This is often due to the immunization of the person with a toxoid or vaccine, leading to the production of antibiotics that are stimulated by immunization. Since immune system is stimulated to produce antibodies that would not have been normally produced naturally, this is viewed as an artificial form of acquired or adaptive immunity.

Passive immunity

Immunity can also be characterized as being passive or active in nature. Passive immunity exists when the person receives antibodies or even transfers T-cells from the outside. Passive immunity can be part of both adaptive or artificial immunity and natural immunity. Furthermore, passive immunity often exists through the transfer of antibodies through breast milk in the young nursing infant. However, probably the most well-known passive immunity happens through the adaptive or artificial level, where an agent such a gamma globulin is injected into the individual. When a person is inoculated on a passive immunity level, the person incurs protection usually instantaneously. However, the protection only lasts for a short duration, often no longer than weeks or a couple of months.

Active immunity

Active immunity provides a much longer duration of protection, and it may provide protection of the individual over his or her entire life. Here again, active immunity can happen both through natural or artificial levels. On a natural level, we often incur immunity through interacting with our environment, encountering common bacterium and viral agents that enter our body and provoke an immune response, often unbeknownst to us.

Active immunity can also occur through the artificial means of obtaining immunizations that stimulate the body's immune system to produce antibodies to the antigenic substance that is introduced into the body. Through the introduction of vaccines of toxoids, the goal is to stimulate the B-cells to produce memory and plasma cells that will ultimately produce antibodies to prepare the body to attack and fight these microbial agents when the body does encounter them.

Humoral immunity and cell-mediated immunity

Finally, immunity can be differentiated into humoral and cell-mediated immunity (Goldberg, 2007). With humoral immunity, the body produces antibodies to counteract the effect of an invading antigenic agent. Antibodies are usually quite specific to the antigen, and when specific antigens enter the body, memory cells initiate specific plasma cells to release the requisite antibodies to attack the antigen.

The cell-mediated form of immunity is initiated by T-cells. These cells often are cytotoxic in the effect. Cell-mediated immunity can be passive, as when T-cells are introduced from the outside into the person's body, or active, when the person's own T-cells, which are part of the endogenous environment of the individual, work to directly attack the antigenic agent, such as a bacteria, virus, fungi, parasitic agent, or even cancer cells. T-cells also release cytokines that attract phagocytes to the location of the infection for further immunologic activity.

Microbes That Cause Infectious Diseases

There are five major types of infectious agents that are often mentioned as being the microbial cause of disease (National Institute of Health Education). These five major categories are bacteria, viruses, fungi, protozoa, and helminths. The National Institute of Health and many microbiologist and infection disease specialists have within the last 30 years become aware of prions, which now are often considered their own separate classification. Although those who work in infection control within healthcare do not have to hold a level of expertise equivalent to a microbiologist, one nevertheless must have some understanding of those microbial agents that are often involved in causing many forms of disease.

Bacteria

Bacteria are unicellular prokaryotic organisms. They are very small, usually measured in micrometers (one millionth of a meter), and can only be seen through the use of a microscope. They also have no organized internal membranous structures, such as mitochondria or golgi apparatus, that are usually clearly articulated and defined in other single cells, known as eukaryotes. They also have a single gene and typically reproduce by binary fission, an asexual splitting of the cell.

Most bacteria have a cell wall on the outside and an inner plasma membrane, although some bacteria only have a plasma membrane. Bacteria often have cell walls with different compositions, which are found chemically, allowing them to be stained in the laboratory. This is often quite useful medically for detailing the level of pathogen that exists, its level of pathogenicity, as well as its susceptibility to certain types of antibiotic treatments. The two major categories of staining classification that often provide a useful indication for pharmacological treatment are referred to as gram positive or gram negative. The more intricate details of the gram staining procedure and its implications are beyond the nature of this book. However, it is helpful to understand and be somewhat conversant with this terminology. There are many other types of staining, such as acid-fast staining found in the tuberculosis bacterium, that are quite useful for medical purposes.

Another very useful way of classifying bacteria, and the one most often referred to, is based on a bacteria's morphology. This deals with how they appear under the microscope. Generally speaking, there are three major classifications with minor variations within each classification. The three major classifications, based on appearance, are cocci, bacillus, and curved. Coccus bacteria, bacterialcoccal, or cocci are spherical in appearance. Often three major types of cocci are referred to: streptococci, staphylococci, and diplococcic. The streptococcus is a bacterium that is spherical and linear, comprise of a number of spheres organized in a straight line. The staphylococcus is a group of spheres that are clumped together, resembling a bunch of grapes. Finally, the diplococcal bacterium is two spheres aligned next to each other in a linear organization. The following is a diagram of the different coccal bacteria discussed (Figure 2.1).

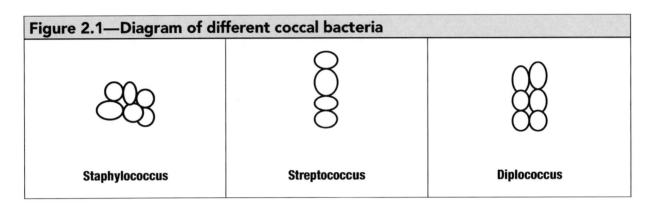

Figure 2.1—Diagram of different coccal bacteria

The second major type of bacteria based on its morphology is the bacillus. They are often referred to as rod bacteria because their segments look like rods, elongated and capsule shaped. Bacilli also come in a number of varieties, but a few of the major bacillus varieties are the single bacillus, the diplobacillus, and the streptobacillus. The single bacillus is a single, elongated, capsular-shaped bacterium. The diplobacillus, similar to the diplococcic, are made up of two fused bacillus segments. Finally, the streptobacillus is made up of a number of elongated segments that are fused together. The following is a diagram of the three major forms of bacillus (Figure 2.2).

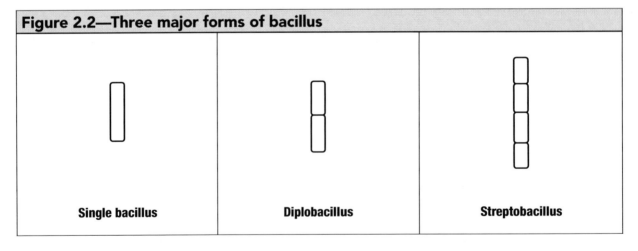

Figure 2.2—Three major forms of bacillus

Finally, the third classification mentioned was the curved type of bacteria. Their morphology is referred to as curved shaped since they do not have the linearity of the bacillus or the spherical features of the cocci. They often are curved, zigzagging forms of bacteria. These bacteria have a number of different variations as well, but the three major variants are the spirochete, the spirillum, and the vibrio. The spirochete looks somewhat like a corkscrew in appearance, such as the bacterium found in syphilis. The spirillum is less frenetically curved than the spirochete; its curves are much smoother. The vibrio, such as those found in cholera, are more comma shaped. The following is a diagram of the three major forms of curved bacteria (Figure 2.3).

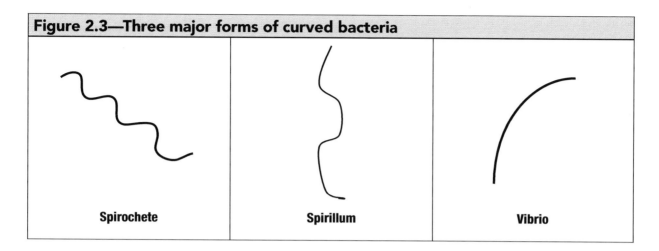

Figure 2.3—Three major forms of curved bacteria

Spirochete   Spirillum   Vibrio

Viruses

A virus is one of the smallest infectious agents that exist. It is much smaller than bacteria and is usually measured in nanometers. A virus is composed of a simple structure. It has no inner cellular structures or membranous features. As such it is composed of a strand of DNA or RNA, which is encased in a protein capsule, the capsid.

The virus, the mature viral particle called a virion, does not have a living structure like other organisms. It does not grow. Nor does it have a type of reproduction pattern that is typically found in other living organisms. Their apparent existence is predicated on replicating and passing on their genetic strands of DNA or RNA. However, it cannot replicate by themselves. They are reliant on being intracellular parasites. In other words, it needs to penetrate living cells and use these cells' nucleic acid or genetic material to continue to manufacture their very existence. Generally speaking, viruses follows the following cycle: First, they attach themselves to the living host cell, such as a human cell, and then penetrate the cell. They direct the replication of further virus particles by using their DNA or RNA as something akin to a master recipe. The viruses' genetic material, the DNA or RNA, uses the host cell and its genetic material and assembles it according to the template of the virus' genetic material. Remember, it is doing all of this inside the human cell, or any living organism's cell, since the virus is an intracellular parasite. After it manufactures the virus using the living host cell's genetic material, the newly assembled virus is then released out of the cell to further infect more cells. Typically, many of the living host cells that have been parasitized by the virus are now weakened or even killed off by the virus's parasitic activity.

Some common viruses found among the elderly within long-term care, frequently due to their immunocompromised status, include:

- **Herpes Zoster:** This is often referred more common as "Shingles." It happens due to a reactivation of the chicken pox virus (varicella virus). It often leads to highly painful blistering skin lesions that often settle over a nerve plexus area.

- **Respiratory Syncytial Virus (RSV):** This paramyxoviridae virus is a virus often associated with young children. It is a respiratory virus that causes significant respiratory issues and can lead to hospitalization. It causes lower respiratory tract infections and is now recognized as an important virus that is found in many long-term care facilities.

- **Other Respiratory Viral Infection due to Influenza:** In addition to RSV, other viral infections related to influenza are commonly found among the elderly. Among these, post-influenza pneumonia is common.

Fungi

Fungi are saprophytic, absorbing nutrients from often dead and decaying matter, and some are parasitic. Some fungi are unicellular, but most are multicellular organisms, having much greater cellular complexity than the previous microorganisms. Fungi share a cell wall with bacteria. However, the composition of the cell wall is much different in fungi. Often, the cell wall is made of cellulose, chitin, and complex polysaccharides. Their major method of reproduction is through the formation of spores.

The makeup of fungi is quite evident under the microscope. For instance, if one looks at a mushroom, a form of fungus, one will see many small filaments. These filaments are called hyphae. When hyphae are combined, they form into a larger structure, the mycelium. Fungi often infiltrate areas by releasing spores, and fungal infections often thrive in moist areas of the body, where, as a saphrophytic agent, it can acclimate itself quite well. Below is an illustration of a mushroom. Notice the fusing hypha and, as the aggregation of hyphae are brought together, the structural mycelium that is able to be seen without a microscope (Figure 2.4).

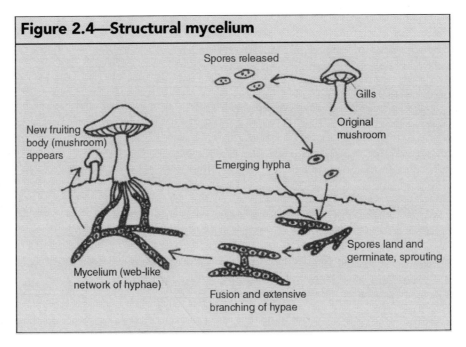

Figure 2.4—Structural mycelium

The pathogenicity of fungi for human diseases can range from negligible, such as that found in edible mushrooms, to highly pathogenic and virulent in their disease-causing ability. The study of fungi is referred to as mycology, and fungal infections frequently are referred to as mycotic infections. Many common mycotic infections in humans can be relatively minor, such as tenia pedis (athlete's foot) and tenia capitis (ringworm in the scalp), tenia, cruris (jock itch), and tenia corporis (ringworm of the skin), to more severe and life-threatening fungal infections such as histoplasmosis, which often settles in the lung, or crytococcol meningitis. A common infection by the genus Candida often leads to candidiasis, a type of vaginal yeast infection in women. The same fungal specimen frequently leads to oral and throat yeast infections (trench mouth or thrush) due to treatment with corticosteroids and the patient being immunocompromised.

Protozoa

Most of us were introduced to protozoa in our middle and high school biology courses. Protozoa are single-celled organisms. Moreover, they have greater complexity than the prokaryotic bacteria organisms. Protozoa are eukaryotes. Therefore, they have membrane-bound organelles on an intracellular level. Protozoans do not have a cell wall; rather, they just have a plasma membrane. They are also quite small, typically smaller than 50 micrometers, but are larger than bacteria and especially larger than viruses. However, microscopic analysis is still needed to examine protozoa.

Protozoa can be acquired through swimming in lakes or rivers, being bitten by arthropods, tcontact with fecal contaminates, or ingestion of contaminated food or water supplies. Malaria, a disease that many have heard of, is transmitted by mosquitos carrying the protozoan organism Plasmodium Vivox. Other diseases of the gastrointestinal tract, such as Giardia Lamblia, cause intestinal discomfort and mucousy stools and diarrhea. Toxoplasmosis, caused by Toxoplasma Gondii, which is a very common parasitic disease, is often spread by cats and cats' feces. A sexually transmitted disease, Trichomoniasis, is caused by the protozoan organism, Trichomonas Vaginalis.

Protozoan organisms are frequently classified by their movement. Mastigophora are flagellates with a whip-like tail involved in their locomotion. Ciliates use hair-like projections that surround their outer membrane to engage in movement. The Sarcodina protozoans move using amoeboid movement, which is referred to as pseudopodia. Sporozoans are protozoa that lack mobility.

Protozoan organisms do not often pose problems, but they can become a primary etiological factor, or even opportunistic, especially among those individuals who are immunocompromised. Furthermore, many protozoans can be difficult to kill. This is due to some protozoa using a protective structure, called a pellicle, which leaves them with a strong outer surface. Others form "tests," a shell made out of calcium carbonate, while other protozoan organisms form "cysts," which are a resting stage with a thick, resistant covering.

Helminths

Helminth is a technical term for a number of different types of worms that can become associated with parasitic infections in human beings. There are a few major classifications of these worms. For instance, platyhelminths is a technical term for the phylum associated with flatworms such as flukes or tapeworms. The phylum Nematoda is made up of various types of roundworms that can also have serious parasitic implications.

Generally speaking, helminths create disease and illness by using a human as a host, parasitizing the human and living within the body. Furthermore, many helminths have complex life cycles in which they pass through several stages of development within the host. Trematoda, or flukes, are all parasitic, and have complex life cycles specialized for parasitism in animal tissues. Many eventually settle in major organs, leading to a potentially fatal impact. For instance, after passing through several stages, the human lung fluke eventually settles in the lung. Another flatworm species, the Schistosoma, leads to Schistosomias, which lives in the blood especially close to the intestinal area, and can lead to extensive damage of the intestines, bladder, and kidneys. Fasciola Hepatica moves through the intestinal wall and parasitizes the liver, causing it to fail. A more familiar disease, trichinosis, is conveyed through eating improperly cooked meat, in particular pork. This disease is caused by the trichinella roundworm, which settles in muscle, heart, and brain tissue, eventually causing death. Other parasitic worms that are fairly common throughout the world are (1) ascaris, a round worm that causes ascariasis and can grow to over a foot long and infect the intestinal area; (2) other forms of hookworms that parasitize the intestinal track; and (3) pinworm infections, the most common of the parasitic worm infections, more frequently found in children and infecting the lower digestive tract, in particular the colon/rectal area.

Other non-helminth parasites

A quick mention should be made of other parasites that may exist and spread through a healthcare facility, leading to infection control issues. Many may not originate within the facility but are brought in by patients, family members, or visitors. Here are a few of the more common ones:

- **Acariasis** (a mite): Acariasis is caused by the acari organism and bedbugs, which are often spread through clothing, bedding, or skin-to-skin contact.
- **Pediculosis humanis** (head lice) and pediculosis humanis corporis (body lice): These are often spread by contact with the hosts head and hair or body.
- **Pediculosis pubis** (pubic crab lice): This is less common among long-term care population, but with younger individuals coming in for more subacute issues, the potential for such infection to be conveyed through contact with a fomite exists.
- **Scabies** (colloquially known as the seven-year itch): This mite tunnels in the skin and causes severe itching and a rash. This has been a frequent parasite that has caused skin problems in many long-term care environments.
- **Human Fleas:** These arthropods live off of the blood of the host, at times causing anemia.

Prions

Very little will be stated about these since very little is still known. At first, when proposed by Stanley Prusiner, who won the Nobel Prize for his work on the prion, it was thought that they were an impossibility. This is because the prion, contrary to all other forms of infectious organisms, is made exclusively out of a protein. It has no nucleic acids, such as DNA or RNA, and the thought of a protein existing without any nucleic acid template was difficult, if not impossible, to fathom. However, it is now thought that many of the devastating diseases once referred to as slow viruses, such as Creuzfeldt-Jakob disease in humans, scrapie in sheep, and bovine spongiform encephalopathy (commonly referred to as "mad cow disease") are now caused by prions. Concern regarding infections due to prions is not a large issue for long-term healthcare professionals at this time.

Control of the Growth of Microbes

Those who work with infection control have to be versed in common strategies used to lessen, minimize, or even eradicate microbial growth. In hospitals, many administrators relegate the infectious disease issues to experts in the area, so the hospital administrator can focus on the day-to-day business. However, long-term care facilities are typically smaller settings without full-time infectious disease specialists on staff, and they don't have in-house labs that can provide quick cultures; because of this, everyone at the facility, including administrators, must be involved in infection control. Staff members in administration, dietary supervisors, laundry and maintenance supervisors, physical and occupational therapists, activity therapists, and nursing staff need to have a working knowledge of key concepts for inhibiting microbial growth, because they are all intricately linked in infection control. Let us examine some major concepts in this area.

In speaking about inhibiting microbial growth some common terms are used. There is often confusion among many of these terms, and they are frequently used incorrectly. The following are some common concepts:

- **Sterilization:** Sterilization is the process of eradicating all microorganisms from an object. Think about sterilization as wiping a slate clean of everything. Perfectly achieved sterile fields are often far less achieved due to its extreme eradication process and methods needed to achieve this process.
- **Disinfection:** Disinfection is the use of a disinfectant, which is a chemical agent that, when applied to an inanimate object or surface, reduces the microbial number and inhibits the microbial growth of potential pathogens. It does not eliminate everything, but it dramatically reduces the threat of disease.
- **Antiseptic:** These are agents that can be administered to the external tissue on the human body to help reduce the potential for infection. Antiseptics are not taken internally, but when applied to the skin, they reduce the risk of microbial infections invading the body.

- **Static versus cidal agents:** A statis agent reduces or inhibits a microorganizm's growth. For instance, a bacteriostatic agent inhibits the growth of potential disease-causing bacterial agents. A cidal agent is one that kills the microorganism. Bactericidal, viricidal, or fungicidal agents are those that kill bacteria, viruses, and fungi.

Before leaving the topic of microbial growth, a couple of methods by which growth can be controlled should be mentioned. Generally speaking, there are two major methods: physical and chemical. Both forms can be highly successful; however, due to the limited amount of resources often found in nursing care centers, chemical methods are often the chief means by which microbial control is done. Nevertheless, a discussion of both will be provided here.

Physical methods provide considerable protection from microbial infection. One of the most well-known types used is heat. Heat provides protection through denaturing proteins. In the human body, many proteins are denatured at approximately 40°C. Another form of heat that has been a standby for years is boiling equipment at 100°C/212°F for 15 minutes, which kills many bacterial and viral agents. Pasteurization, which uses much lower temperatures, works similarly to provide healthy food to consumers.

Autoclaving, a combination system that uses moist heat and pressure (typically 121.5°C at 15 psi for 15 minutes), is one of the best ways to kill microbes. Autoclaves are not inexpoensive, so many nursing homes often don't have them. Desiccation, which uses very low temperatures to kill microbes, using ultraviolet radiation, and using ionizing radiation (such as alpha, beta, gamma, or x rays) can be highly effective at killing microbes and providing sterilization. However, most of these methods are not used in nursing homes due to the cost, the special resources needed, and the specific professionals that would need to be employed.

Chemical methods are the most commonly used within long-term care environments. While there are many chemical methods that can be used, only a few of the more common methods will be mentioned here. One of the most powerful, introduced by Joseph Lister: phenols. Phenols are benzene rings with an OH molecule and cresols, which are phenols with a methane molecule. Many are very powerful substances. They are toxic and disrupt the cellular membrane of the microorganism and lead to protein denaturing. Lysol is a common phenol.

Halogens, named after where they fall on the periodic table of elements, are also commonly used for microbial control. Iodine, chlorine, and fluorine are common halogens. Fluorine is probably most recognized for its dental uses. Iodine is commonly found in tinctures used on cuts, as an antiseptic agent, or to disinfect an area. Chlorine is a strong oxidizing agent found in many bleach preparations.

Alcohols are also commonly used for microbial control. The two most commonly used alcohol preparations are isopropyl and ethyl alcohol. They evaporate quickly, so surfaces requiring more time to kill microbes may need to use something other than alcohol. However, alcohol, because it evaporates quickly, is often preferred as a skin antiseptic for injection areas.

Soaps and detergents are often a first-line level of control for microbial control. Washing one's hands using soap and water is often the most effective way to prevent the spread of disease. Soap and detergents do not have any mystical properties. They are surfactants, lowering the surface tension of the microbes to the surface, which allows them to be removed. Detergents act in the same way as well. Many detergents, called quaternary ammonium compound (quats), are used in the dietary area for dish and utensil washing. In addition, many of these soaps and detergents have emulsifiers, carrying away oils that may also harbor microorganisms.

Oxidizing agents have briefly been mentioned with chlorine. However, other common microbial oxidizers are hydrogen peroxide, benzoyl peroxide, and ozone. All release large amounts of oxygen, which is highly toxic and catabolic to microorganisms. In fact, excessive oxidizing agents in the human body can be toxic and have destructive effects on human body tissue, regardless of any microbial influence.

There are many other types of physical and chemical methods that could be mentioned. However, the purpose of this book is to acquaint the reader with some important aspects of infection control and not be an exhaustive compendium, listing all of the methods that can be used for microbial control. What has been listed here should suffice to provide the long-term care worker with a working knowledge of microbe growth control.

Antibiotic Resistance and Antibiotic Stewardship

Antibiotic resistance is a growing problem. Today, due too often to healthcare's cursory and injudicious use of antibiotics, for conditions that antibiotics are not useful for, many bacterial infections no longer respond to antibiotics or the antibiotic's effects have been attenuated. This has caused many problems.

First, many formerly susceptible bacteria are now resistant to antibiotics. While there was a broad spectrum of antibiotics that worked on many bacterial organisms, that spectrum has shrunk considerably. Even more problematic is the number of microbes that are resistant to everything in our antibiotic arsenal, including our strongest antibiotics.

Another issue is that bacteria and their genetics are proving to be smarter than humans. Since we have abused the use of antibiotics, these small, microscopic agents have adapted on an evolutionary level to outsmart us, creating a genomic resistance on the microbial level toward our high technology pharmaceutical arsenal of antibiotics, which were once believed to be wonder drugs. Penicillin or a sulfonamide can no longer wipe out a number of genus and species of bacterium. These small microbes are telling us that we had our way much too long and now we must adapt to them.

Although pharmaceutical companies have heard the bacterial union representative loud and clear saying we must adapt to them, in reality, finding new antibiotics is often quite expensive and difficult. One single antibiotic which was able to efficaciously wipe out a large number of microbes is more difficult to pharmacologically produce due to the level of resistance that has developed. Today, many antibiotics are targeted toward addressing more specific microbes and, therefore, come to market with fewer benefits and more levels of microbial specificity.

Now that microbes have become antibiotic resistant, their momentum is hard to stop. Our ability to introduce new antibiotics is being outpaced by the snowballing numbers of microbes developing antibiotic resistance. Even with the new drugs that are coming to market, the duration of their efficacy is often not known due to the changing bacterial genetics that has led these little microscopic entities to develop resistance at an accelerating rate.

In 2013, the CDC evaluated the threat of this problem by classifying 18 forms of microorganisms that are of important concern (*http://www.cdc.gov/drugresistance/biggest_threats.html*). In fact, they went on to place these microorganisms and their levels of resistance into three categories based on the CDC's level of perceived threat. These categories are: urgent, serious, and concerning. Those classified as urgent or serious need to have immediate attention. Those classified as concerning, although needing less immediate surveillance, still need to be monitored closely so they do not become urgent and serious threats. The following are the microorganisms that they listed according to the categories mentioned:

Urgent Classification

- **Clostridium Difficile** (Cdiff): This is a very common microorganism found in long-term care settings that causes severe intestinal infections and can be life-threatening

- **Carbapenem-Resistant Enterobacteriaceae**: This bacteria has developed an antibiotic resistance that leaves it life-threatening

- **Neisseria gonorrhoeae**: While once fairly easily treated, this organism responsible for the sexually trans-mitted disease, has mutated and become increasingly antibiotic resistant

Serious Classification

- Multidrug-Resistant Acinetobacter
- Drug-Resistant Campylobacter
- Fluconazole-Resistant Candida: This yeast infection, often viewed as potentially innocuous, is now the fourth leading cause of blood stream infections in healthcare facilities
- Extended Spectrum Enterobacteriaceae (ESBL)
- Vancomycin-Resistant Enterococcus (VRE): VRE is now resistant to our most powerful antibiotic
- Multidrug-Resistant Pseudomonas Aeruginosa: Often an opportunistic agent, it now has multiple antimicrobial levels of resistance
- Drug-Resistant Non-Typhoidal Salmonella
- Drug-Resistant Salmonella Serotype Typhi
- Drug-Resistant Shigella
- Methicillin-Resistant Staphylococcus Aureus (MRSA): On the healthcare radar for some time now, MRSA has caused many deaths due to its resistance and is a frequent organism found in long-term care environments
- Drug-Resistant Streptococcus Pneumoniae: A leading cause of pneumonia, this is a common problem among many sedentary and bed-bound residents in long-term care
- Drug-Resistant Tuberculosis

Concerning Classification

- Vancomycin-Resistant Staphylococcus Aureus: Once contracted is even more problematic than MRSA, since now it is resistant to the most potent drug in our arsenal
- Erythromycin-Resistant Group A Streptococcus: This causes strep throat, toxic shock syndrome, necrotizing fasciitis, and impetigo, just to name a few
- Clindamycin-Resistant Group B Streptococcus

Excessive and inappropriate use of antibiotics has led to bacterial resistance. This is not to say that even if antibiotics were used consistently and judiciously antibacterial resistance would not have happened. Microorganisms are "smart" in the adaptive and evolutionary sense, so even under ideal conditions, antibiotic exposure would have led to microorganisms adapting genetically; resistance would always come to exist in some manner. However, our failure to use antibiotics in a prudent manner, for infections that they are targeted toward addressing, has led to a current problem of antimicrobial resistance that is outpacing our ability to devise and manufacture new medications to keep up with the runaway problem. Again, although this book is dealing with infection control in long-term care, its impact extends well beyond that realm and is a problem that has become a world-wide public health issue.

The urgent and serious catergorization of the diseases and antimicrobial resistance mentioned above, coupled with the increasing the CDC has for a number of other microbes and diseases becoming resistant has caused the CDC to call for instituting an "antimicrobial stewardship" program within healthcare settings to help slow down or reduce the growing problem in this area. According to the CDC, antimicrobial stewardship programs should encompass the following (*http://www.cdc.gov/getsmart/healthcare/implementation/core-elements.html*):

- A leadership commitment that dedicates the "necessary human, financial, and information technology resources" must exist.
- Accountability needs to be developed in the program, often through a single leader who is responsible for program outcomes.

- A person with drug expertise, in particular a pharmacist, needs to be appointed to enhance appropriate antibiotic use. For most long-term care facilities, this would typically be the consulting pharmacist the long-term care facility uses to do their pharmaceutical audits.

- The CDC advises utilizing an "action" to be tied to systemic evaluation of antibiotic therapy and consistent "tracking," which monitors how and for what reason antibiotics are prescribed, as well as the development of any resistance patterns that appear to be found in the healthcare facility.

- Providing regular reports on the antibiotic use and resistance within the healthcare facility to physicians, nurses, and all relevant staff is necessary.

- Continually educating clinicians on resistance and optimal methods of prescribing antimicrobial therapy is necessary to help reinforce the importance and pervasive nature of this issue.

Bodily Defense Against Disease

The human body, the host for various microbial organisms, tends to become more susceptible to disease as it ages. Since many nursing care centers have large populations of older adults, one can see how they become particularly susceptible environments for disease. In addition to their age, many individuals in nursing care centers already have diseases that stress their immune system. This increases the susceptibility toward disease among individuals in this environment.

Understanding the importance of the body's immune system, the system that individuals have to fight disease, as it relates to infection control is important. As was stated, whether you are an administrator, medical director, director of nursing, staff nurse or nurse assistant, physical therapist, activity director, dietician or dietary personnel, or maintenance director, if you work in this environment, you are constantly going to be interfacing with a population that will have varying levels of disease susceptibility. Furthermore, you will also be working within a population that has varying levels of resistance, or the ability to ward off disease. Understanding the population you are working with and these two important concepts of susceptibility and resistance as they relate to your healthcare organization's population, plays a paramount role in infection control.

People have two types of immunity: "natural" and "adaptive." These systems are the first line of mechanisms that protect us against disease. Their complexity is well beyond the scope of this book. However, a basic understanding of some major concepts regarding the immune system does need to be understood, especially since the core features of infection control are based on these concepts.

Natural immune system

Natural defenses are classified as "innate" or "nonspecific." We are born with many natural defenses that guard us against all forms of infectious agents, not just one or a few things in particular.

The most important nonspecific natural defense is the largest organ in the human body: skin. The skin forms an outer protective mechanism. Skin that is intact is often impermeable to most forms of infectious agents. When compromised skin leaves a "portal of entry" for microorganisms to enter the body. Additionally, as individuals age, skin integrity is often compromised, becoming thinner and easily torn. Therefore, due to the compromised skin issues that are often part of this population, this can lead to an important issue for microbial infection. Most may not think of skin care issues and training in skin care as having anything to do with infection control, but since skin loses its elasticity and normal turgor and integrity as one ages, addressing resident skin issues that may further compromise their resistance needs to be done promptly and skillfully.

In addition to the skin being a formidable barrier to microorganisms, the skin related surfaces often provide other mechanisms to fight disease. For instance, immunoglobulin A, which is found in many secretions, plays a first line role in fighting microorganisms. Mucous membranes produce lysozymes. Lysozymes are found in tears, mucous, and saliva. These disease-fighting agents attach to the bacterial cell wall, destroying the microorganism. The lysozymic agents found in a person's secretions may be compromised in older adults, and secretions may become reduced as well, further increasing their susceptibility to disease.

The body also has other natural defenses. The skin again has Langerhans cells that help to take microbial agents and move them to the lymph nodes, helping to establish artificial immunity. The stomach has hydrochloric acid and many enzymes that work at a low pH, which help kill ingested microbes. Oil glands help to provide a protective excretion that defends against infectious agents. We even have cilia, hair-like structures in our nasal passages and throat, to help eliminate potentially harmful particulate matter.

The inflammatory response is another very important natural defense. Although inflammation can be a problem, it has important protective features that can aid in our body's defense. The inflammatory response is actually made up of a number of features: heat, redness, swelling, pain, and often loss of function. Inflammation is the result of cellular damage. As such, inflammation leads to increased heat, redness, and swelling that helps bring our important bodily defense cells, such as neurophils and macrophages, to the site of infection and address, as well as neutralize, the enemy. Pain is also crucial, because it makes us aware of the need to address the issue.

Let us examine some of the important cells that make up our body's soldiers that help fight and provide us with resident disease fighters. Again, since the book is focusing on infection control, the cells mentioned here are far from being an exhaustive enumeration of our internal immune system's defenses. That being stated, even the most rudimentary discussion on immunity has to mention the most common white blood cells leading the charge. These are neutrophils. These individual blood cells are often the first responders, and, of the major white blood cells, they are most numerous. They are predominately phagocytic, a term that means "cell eater." Neutrophils are the most abundant of white blood cells and are often the first responders to infectious agents, moving to the site of infection to help prevent further spread of infection. Neutrophils do not have a long life. They only live one to two days. However, as sentinels, they are always on the lookout for inflammatory areas, and they move quickly from the blood stream to the source of inflammation.

Monocytes are precursors to macrophage cells. Macrophages (meaning "big eaters") often work in collaboration with neutrophils. They can secrete enzymes that are toxic to bacteria, and they then ingest the remnants of the bacterial organisms. Macrophages are highly important for phagocytic activity in our body. Furthermore, they also play a role in helping to sensitize cells in the artificial immune system.

Basophils and mast cells are similar in their function. Basophils are one of the major categories of white blood cells that move in and out of the blood stream. Mast cells are more fixed and found in most tissue, especially located close to blood vessels and mucous membranes. Both are very critical during contact with particular allergens, setting up an allergic response. These are the cells that often are responsible for many of the allergic responses that we take antihistamines for. Why? One of their effects is to secrete histamines, serotonin and heparin, leading to greater blood vessel permeability. The antihistamines often attempt to shrink the tissue inflammation response that causes many types of discomfort.

Eosinophils are the next major type of white blood cell. These cells specialize in dealing with parasites. The number of these white blood cells is quite small in comparison to others. They probably remain as remnants of past evolutionary stages, when hominids experienced greater parasitic contact. Still today in many less developed parts of the world parasitic infections are quite prevalent among individuals.

The above elements that have been discussed are part of the natural or innate defense system of the human body. As such, these defense features are part of us from birth. The white blood cells mentioned do not have the level of specificity as those cells that are found in the more evolutionarily advanced adaptive immune system. They arise from a different lineage of cells, often referred to as myeloid cells and follow this myeloid lineage in their development. The next group of immune cells that will be discussed are part of the more evolutionary advanced adaptive immune system.

Adaptive immune system

The adaptive immune system is composed of predominately the B and T cells. Natural killer cells (NK cells) can fit into this category as well based on their lineage, but they are often quite different from the B and T cells. All these cells arise from a lymphoid stem cell lineage and are a type of white blood cell called lymphocytes. B and T cells are further differentiated in the lymph tissue, giving them greater justification to being referred to as lymphocytes. Animals and plants all have varying levels of natural or innate immunity. However, only higher level animal species, often known as chordates (fish, amphibians, reptiles, and mammals) have evolved the more advanced level of adaptive immunity.

Although NK cells are part of this lineage, many of the similarities to other adaptive immunity cells do not exist. For instance, adaptive immunity is based upon cells changing their genetic makeup when they come into contact with different antigenic agents. NK cells do not do this NK cells have a more general type of defense. Since they do not change their genetic material they maintain a more generalized, yet highly important, response to such things as viruses and even cancer cells. Therefore, their importance toward fighting disease cannot be minimized.

Both B and T cells are more specific in their defenses, and the specificity they develop is the result of the alternation in their genetic makeup as they come into contact with antigens that are potentially disease-causing agents. I will only discuss general features of B and T cells. In reality, there are many subcategories of each, and the delineation of such is far beyond the scope of this book.

B-cells derive bone marrow. B-cells often produce humoral immunity, which means they circulate in the humor, or blood and blood plasma components. These cells differentiate into plasma cells, which secrete antibodies and memory cells and are anamnestic, meaning they are cells that remember specific enemies they encounter, so when encountered again, they can direct a quicker immune response.

Remember that B and T cells are part of adaptive immunity, so they alter their genetic makeup to respond to specific antigenic agents. Plasma cells, or for that matter memory cells, as well, are very specific in their response to antigens. Plasma cells often give humoral immunity its name in that these cells release specific antibodies into the blood to attack the antigens or enemies that reside within the body. However, it is interesting that although plasma cells release antibodies into the blood, they predominately spend most of their time in lymph tissue and only move into the blood stream and release their antibodies when needed.

The major type of antibody groups that exist are called isotypes, or, more technically, immunoglobulins. An immunoglobulin many are familiar with immunoglobulin G, frequently referred to as gamma globulin. Let me briefly mention the five major immunoglobulins:

1. **IgM:** This is often the first responder to infectious agents. As such, the response to infectious agents is slower since memory cells to new antigens have not been acquired.

2. **IgG:** This well-known immunoglobulin is prominent in secondary responses. After memory cells have been acquired, the IgG allows for a much quicker response to the already coded and recognized antigenic agent.

3. **IgA:** Many secretions, especially those on the skin and mucous membranes have protective effects, one reason is because IgA provides your body with this frontline protection.

4. **IgE:** This is prominent in allergies and parasitic infestations. Parasites and allergens cause this agent to bind to eosinophils, basophils, and mast cells, leading to their subsequent measures to deal with antigens.

5. **IgD:** This is much less specific than the other four and acts as an antigenic receptor on B cells.

The other major form of adaptive immunity that will be discussed in this chapter is what is often referred to as cell-mediated immunity. In contrast to the plasma cells that release antibodies to address the antigens, in cell-mediated immunity the lymphocytes come into direct contact with the infectious agent that needs to be destroyed. The major player in cell-mediated immunity is the T cell, of which there are many, but for our discussion we will keep it simple.

Where B cells originate and are differentiated in the bone marrow, T cells migrate to the Thymus gland for differentiation. Therefore, T cell stands for thymus-derived cell. Where B cells express their antibodies within the humoral medium, the blood, to target antigens, T cells come into contact with cells that are often invaded by antigenic agents such as viruses and certain bacteria, thereby poking holes and destroying the cells and the antigenic agents. T cells of this type, referred to as cytotoxic T cells or CD8 cells, are those that conduct this type of duty.

However, there is another very important T cell. It is the helper T cell or (Th cell). It is also referred to as the CD4 cell. Helper T cells are extremely important for coordinating much of the activity of adaptive immunity. This is the cell that is attacked by the HIV virus that can severely compromise the immune system, potentially leading to the death of individual who becomes vulnerable to opportunistic infectious agents. Typically, macrophages present antigens to helper T cells, leading to cellular communication and the promotion of B cell antibody secretion. Helper T cells also help to coordinate memory cells for quicker responses to antigens. Upon contact with an antigen it helps secrete interleukin to stimulate CD8 cells and memory cells. It also helps to initiate the secretion of interferon, putting cells on high alert to protect themselves against specific viruses. Helper T cells even help to make sure the immune system does not overreact by leading T suppressor cells to "call of the dogs off."

This was a brief discussion of the immune system. However, in discussing infection control, one has to have some basic knowledge of immunity, because both are intricately linked. It must be reiterated that even a single immune response encompasses many more immune concepts and actions than were discussed here. However, this brief overview is a foundation to build on and help us move forward in our more specific discussion about infection control.

The 12-Step CDC Program

The CDC has developed a 12-step program for addressing antimicrobial resistance in healthcare settings. Since antimicrobial resistance to many antibiotics has become an increasing concern in long-term care, as well as in society in general, the advisory council for the CDC has come up with important suggestions for dealing with amazingly adaptive and resistant microorganisms. It is important for administrators to understand the importance of addressing this problem.

Step 1: Vaccinate

According to the CDC, prevention is one of the most important steps in dealing with antimicrobial resistance. The CDC encourages vaccination as the critical first step in addressing this problem. Providing vaccinations for influenza and pneumococcal infections to residents and staff members is an important preventive measure. Vaccinations prevent unnecessary illness and transmission of illness, as well as the unnecessary use of antibiotic agents, which has led to the current problem of antimicrobial resistance. Although many individuals take these infections and their vaccinations lightly, vaccinations can be lifesaving, especially among the older adult population. Healthcare workers are encouraged to get the hepatitis B vaccine, and all individuals are encouraged to get a tetanus booster every 10 years.

Step 2: Prevent infections

Preventing conditions that lead to infections is the second step. Recommendations include preventing aspiration, preventing pressure ulcers, and maintaining hydration.

To prevent aspiration, you need to: make sure residents can swallow properly; make sure their dentures fit properly, they are wearing their dentures while they're eating, and they can chew the foods they're eating; make sure the head of the bed is up while a resident is eating or if the resident is on a feeding tube; monitor for proper placement of feeding tubes before each meal; and ensure that the resident does not have gastric regurgitation issues that could lead to aspiration. By paying close attention to these issues, you can prevent food particles from entering the lungs and causing pneumonia.

Preventing pressure ulcers is important because skin is a first line of defense against infections. Any breach in the skin can allow microorganisms to enter the body, so good preventive skin care that impedes skin breakdown is necessary. Furthermore, preventing any further breakdown in the skin once there is a breach in its integrity can prevent unnecessary infections. As pressure ulcers become deeper and larger in scope (going from stage one to stage two, three, or four), the chances of microorganism invasion increase. That is why preventing further degradation of tissue once a pressure ulcer has appeared is very important for infection control.

Maintaining adequate fluid hydration is important for the entire human organism. It helps to filter out bacterial agents and prevent urinary tract infections. It also helps to maintain good skin integrity and provides proper fluid balance in the body, which, if not preserved, can lead to many other issues.

Step 3: Remove unnecessary invasive elements

Eliminating unnecessary use of Foley catheters is the next step. Because Foley catheters are invasive elements that go into the urethra and the bladder, people with Foley catheters in place face higher rates of urinary tract infections. Just inserting a catheter raises the potential for introducing a microorganism into the body. Although this process should follow sterile procedures, there are no guarantees. The longer a catheter is kept in, the greater the likelihood for infection. Therefore, Foley catheters should be used only when absolutely necessary. In fact, catheters are often the leading cause of hospital-acquired infections, and when nursing homes receive patients with catheters, they may already have a pre-existing infection (MARR, 2008).

Other invasive elements, such as parenteral and enteral devices including NG tubes, J-tubes, and even IVs, can also be sites for infection. Therefore, it is important to closely monitor these devices and get rid of them as soon as they are no longer needed to prevent potential infection.

Step 4: Use established criteria

This step concerns using established criteria for diagnosis of infection. Understanding the need to use cultures to identify the type of organism causing a problem and understanding the sensitivity of the organism to particular antibiotic therapy is important. Physicians frequently prescribe a broad-spectrum antibiotic that covers many organisms they anticipate are causing a problem. However, today fewer antibiotics are truly as "broad-spectrum" as they used to be. With bacterial agents modifying their DNA to become resistant to many forms of therapeutic intervention, the general empiric therapy of antibiotic intervention may not be as sound a practice as it once was: the microbe may fail to be sensitive to the chemical agent, and introducing antibiotics that may not be useful for fighting an infection will give other bacteria a greater ability to form further resistance.

Step 5: Know the bugs in your community

Antibiotic resistance is not a homogeneous feature found uniformly in all communities (MARR, 2008). Individuals in different communities also demonstrate different levels of resistance. Although there are many similarities, patterns of infection, antibiotic use, and intervention lead to this deferential in antibiotic resistance. Therefore, it is important to know the bugs in your community. You can do this in a few ways:

- Rely on the local experts in infectious disease control. Providing information to your community health agency and obtaining information from them is important. Complicated infections, which are difficult to cure, rely on an infectious disease expert for advice.

- If residents come to your facility from other facilities or hospitals, make sure you obtain their laboratory results. This allows you to anticipate issues with these residents, especially as they relate to potential resistance.

It is also important for the facility to create its own tracking process. One way to track data on antibiotic resistance is to use an antibiogram (MARR ,2008). An antibiogram tracks resistance over a period of time, typically one year. It examines the data from the bacterial isolates that are received from laboratory reports in relation to the culture and sensitivity results of the antibiotics used and found to be sensitive or not sensitive to the particular organism. It also calculates the percentage of resistance that was found for each organism as it relates to the antimicrobial agents used. This can be valuable for understanding the types of organisms commonly found in your facility and the level of resistance you are dealing with. It also enables the medical director and facility physicians to tailor their therapy. For instance, if you knew that 75% of the E. coli infections in your facility were susceptible to Pen VK, you'd know that 25% coming into your facility were resistant to this antimicrobial intervention.

Step 6: Use antimicrobials wisely

Using antimicrobials wisely is the sixth step. In other words, know when to say no. Estimates show that a whopping 50%–60% of internal, systemic antimicrobials and approximately 60% of topical antibiotic agents are used inappropriately (MARR 2008). That's a lot of misused drugs, which also leads to a costly waste of medication.

Bacterial agents are smart, which has led to their survival. They existed long before humans arrived on the scene and will probably continue to survive after humans are gone. They are resilient organisms that have continued to exist because they have adapted to all forms of environments. Their speed of adaptation to antibiotic agents far exceeds our ability to make new antibiotics. As we continue to use more antibiotics, their ability to adjust their genetic information to become resistant toward these drugs makes them the most formidable opponent that humans have ever faced. Therefore, the CDC recommends judicious use of antibiotic therapy that appropriately targets the organisms susceptible to antimicrobial intervention.

Step 7: Treat infection

This step advises you to treat infection, not colonization or contamination. Many forms of resistant bacteria become colonized and remain in the body without causing any problems. Furthermore, just because a person has encountered some level of contamination does not mean they need an antibiotic prophylaxis. The body has its own system of defense. Even among the elderly, the body is often able to fight off infectious agents on its own.

Therefore, it is important to use proper treatment targeted toward the specific agent that is causing the infection— if the body needs assistance fighting the infection. If symptoms fail to exist, there is often no reason to introduce an agent that may cause side effects and lead to further microbial resistance. According to the CDC, when treatment is needed, it should be reevaluated every 48–72 hours.

Step 8: Stop antimicrobial treatment

When cultures are negative and infection is unlikely, there is no need to introduce antimicrobial therapy; doing so will lead to further microbial adaptation and resistance. Also, when an infection has resolved itself and the course of antimicrobial therapy has been completed, cultures typically are not needed if symptoms have abated.

Step 9: Isolate the pathogen

The pathogen is the disease-causing organism. One way to prevent the spread of drug-resistant microorganisms is to isolate them and not cross-contaminate others with the same organism. Proper hand washing is the single most important means of preventing the spread of infection. Furthermore, using universal precautions, whereby you treat all residents and their body fluids as though they harbored infectious agents, regardless of their diagnoses, is very important in preventing the spread of antibiotic-resistant germs that may be transferred to others, as is using personal protective equipment (especially gloves, gowns, or masks), when providing care. Employees should wash their hands even when using personal protective equipment, and they should wash their hands before and after they provide care for a resident. In addition, potentially infectious agents, such as gloves, should be disposed of properly and promptly.

Sometimes you may need to isolate a person because they are infected with a highly communicable and infectious pathogen. If an individual needs single-room isolation, he or she should be placed in a room designed for this, such as a negative-pressure room. Furthermore, many individuals who are not colonized for resistant microorganisms and are potentially actively infectious should be cohort-segregated, meaning they should be placed in a room with another person infected with a similar resistant agent.

Step 10: Break the chain of contagion

The chain for the transmission of an infectious agent requires a source, a person who is susceptible to the infectious microbe, and a method of transmission (MARR, 2008). Stopping the chain of events at the source is important. One way to do this is through hand washing. However, preventing those who are sick from coming to work is another important method. Employers need not encourage workers to stay home with trivial complaints, but if the individual is sick with a potentially communicable illness, he or she should be encouraged to stay home. Furthermore, if you note that an individual appears ill during work hours, you should send the individual home to prevent transmission.

It is also important to educate family members and other visitors to wash their hands, cover their mouths when coughing, and not come in to the facility if they have an infectious illness. Use of alcohol-based solutions is also recommended for staff members and family members. They should be aware that if they touch an area that may harbor considerable levels of microbial agents, such as their mouths, of even inanimate elements that may carry pathogens often referred to as fomites, they should wash their hands or use an alcohol-based solution.

Step 11: Wash your hands properly

Hand washing is probably the best way to prevent unnecessary transmission of potential pathogens, and using proper hand washing technique is key.

To wash your hands properly, wet your hands with warm water, apply soap (which acts as a surfactant), and cleanse all areas of your hands for at least 20 seconds. Hands should be washed on both sides, between the fingers, and at the fingertips. Shorter nails should be encouraged, because long nails harbor bacteria that can be missed during hand washing. When drying your hands, make sure you have a paper towel ready so you don't have to touch the paper towel dispenser. After you wipe your hands dry, use the paper towel to turn off the sink if it does not have foot controls.

Family members and residents should also be educated on proper hand washing techniques. If residents cannot wash their own hands, staff members should wash residents' hands before and after they eat, as well as throughout the day. The goal here is not to encourage a person to become an obsessive-compulsive hand washer or to develop a germ phobia; it is to use the most primary means for preventing infections.

Step 12: Identify residents with multidrug-resistant organisms (MDROs)

It is important to develop a surveillance program that identifies both new admissions and existing residents who harbor MDROs. Usually the person to develop the program is the one who tracks infections in the building. Often this requires diligence. Examining cultures as they arrive and having other nurses work with infection control personnel to relay information regarding cultured specimens that are identified to be multidrug-resistant will help the infection control person or team keep a running tab of the type of organism and its specific resistance.

The mode of acquisition of the infection should also be tracked. Three common modes of acquisition exist (MARR, 2008):

- **Nosocomial:** Nosocomial means healthcare-acquired. Nosocomial infections are infections the resident picks up in the healthcare facility.

- **Healthcare-associated:** These are infections a resident picks up due to a healthcare procedure. For instance, an IV placed in a resident could cause an infection at the site, which leads to sepsis. These are sometimes also viewed as nosocomial infections, but using the "healthcare-associated" category brings greater specificity to the definition. Healthcare workers who catch an infection while providing care to residents would fit into this category as well.

- **Community-associated:** This type of infection results from patients/residents acquiring an illness within the community, not due to the healthcare they received or the healthcare facility they were in. For instance, a resident may go home for a visit and catch the flu from an ill family member.

The person responsible for identifying MDROs has to track down this information, document the isolated microbe, determine the percent sensitivity and percent resistance to an antibiotic, and calculate infection rates and incidence rates. To calculate an individual's infection rate, use this formula (MARR, 2008, Chapter 12):

$$\text{Individual infection rate} = \frac{X}{Y} \times K$$

where:

- X = The number of individual cases meeting a particular criterion
- Y = The number of residents or resident days of experiencing the particular event or infection

The results of the division are multiplied by K, which is a constant, often expressed as 100. This puts it in percentage form.

Other rates, such as the incidence (the rate of new infections within a given period of time), and prevalence (the total or actual number of cases of disease that currently exist) are important as well.

Proper surveillance of MDROs provides a fruitful level of information for treating and preventing further infections. You cannot cure the problem of drug resistance, but if you address the issue in a judicious manner, you can control it.

Chapter 3

Discussing Some Crucial and Often Overlooked Areas

Although much weight in infection control is given to direct worker-to-resident or patient contact in healthcare settings, throughout this book, references will be made to linen, food, and eating. These areas need to be addressed more specifically before we leave this chapter since infection control is a ubiquitous issue. What follows is a greater explication of these areas that are often overlooked as they relate to properly controlling infections.

Infection Control in the Dietary Area

Although infection control is often given great attention in the nursing area, the dietary area, and its interaction with the infection control program, should be given more attention. Residents in skilled nursing care environments, often have varying degrees of immunocompromised status. Because of this, controlling the potentially invasive impact of food and dietary infection is as important as following sterile procedure for placement of an IV.

One of the first things an administrator needs to understand is which factors make food potentially hazardous and how to guard against these problems. First, acidic products and the pH of food are very important. Foods that have a lower pH, meaning they are more acidic, inhibit bacterial growth. Foods such as oranges, tomatoes, and vinegar have a low pH, and thus are quite acidic. A pH that is less than 4.6 often inhibits the growth of potentially pathogenic organisms (Thomson Prometic, 2005).

Another major area that must be monitored for potentially hazardous food-borne illnesses is the food's water activity, which is measured on a scale. Food water activity, abbreviated a_w, refers to water in food that is not bound to the food molecules. The higher the a_w, the greater the likelihood for pathogenic growth from bacteria, yeasts, or molds. Foods with an a_w of 0.85 or higher are more likely to allow pathogenic organisms to grow and potentially infect individuals. Most foods have a water activity level that is higher than 0.85, but some foods, such as coffee and cookies, have an a_w that is only in the 0.2–0.3 range and hold low potential for growth.

By monitoring the acidity and water activity of the food, a facility can control food spoilage and prevent residents from acquiring food-borne illnesses. Therefore, administrators and their dietary managers must understand these concepts. Although administrators are not directly involved with dietary concerns on a daily basis, their knowledge of these concepts is very important.

Canned and dry food

Canned and vacuum-packed foods should be inspected upon receipt and use. Clostridium botulinum can grow in both types of food products. Instruct your employees that if a can is swollen or bulging, they should not open the can; if they do, they can spread botulism, which is very toxic in small amounts. If your facility receives a shipment of canned goods that is in this condition, the facility should not accept it. In addition, instruct employees that if they push on one end of the can and it causes the other end to make a popping sound, they should not open the can or they should reject the shipment. The same holds true for cans that are leaking or not adequately sealed or labeled. Although it is not the administrator's job to check canned goods for this problem, the administrator should have knowledge of the issue so that he or she can question whether the kitchen staff is following this protocol (Thomson Company, 2005).

Storage is very important as well. Store all dry foods and cans at least 6 inches above floor level. The storage area should be clean and tidy. Keep storage doors closed to prevent further forms of contamination. This is an important area for administrators to inspect during rounds.

Cooling, thawing, and reheating

Proper procedure for cooling, thawing, and reheating food is necessary to prevent food-borne illnesses. Although many individuals will just leave food out to cool, food professionals have outlined a specific protocol that must be followed:

- **Cooling:** All refrigerated food must be at or below 41°F. However, just because the refrigerator temperature is 41°F does not mean this is the optimal refrigeration temperature for all food. After refrigerated food is cooked, it should follow a six-hour cooling-down process. Within the first two hours, the food should be cooled down to 70°F. Then, before being refrigerated again, it should continue to be cooled down to less than 41°F within four hours.

- **Reheating:** Potentially hazardous food that has been previously cooked and refrigerated must be reheated to a temperature of at least 165°F for 15 seconds. The reheating process should occur as quickly as possible, but it should not take longer than two hours to reach the 165°F standard. A microwave can be used to reheat the food, but it must have a rotating accessory to make sure it is heated to 165°F evenly. Steam tables are not acceptable for reheating food.

- **Thawing:** Frozen foods must be kept at a temperature of 0°F or lower. Frozen food is often thawed at room temperature, but should not be. Food professionals state that the proper way to thaw food is to place the frozen food in the refrigerator and let it thaw gradually; alternatively, you can run the frozen food under cool water that does not exceed 70°F. Furthermore, thawed food products should not exceed 41°F for more than four hours.

Handling, food protection, and monitoring

Temperatures in freezers and refrigerators should be monitored each day on each shift in the dietary department. The best time to take temperatures is when the freezer or refrigerator has not been used for a while. That way, you can ascertain whether an adequate seal exists, preventing the exchange of warm and cool air. Thermometers with glass stems should not be used. It is important to remember that the temperature for refrigerators should not exceed 41°F and freezers should be set at 0°F or lower. These temperatures should be charted for each shift. The same procedure for checking temperatures should apply to refrigerators on the nursing units that contain biologicals or food products.

Ice is a food product that is very important in long-term care. Those who obtain ice should do so following proper hand washing and glove use, especially if the ice comes from an open, rather than closed, dispenser. Furthermore, not everyone should have access to ice. Only those who have been trained in proper handling of ice and food products should have access. Bacteria can still live in frozen conditions.

The danger zone for food products and bacterial growth is 41°F to 135°F. Hot food coming off the tray line should be at least 140°F. Although the FDA code for food preparation provides minimum heating temperatures and times, as a general rule of thumb, heating food to 165°F for at least 15 seconds is a good guide. Monitoring the danger zones and knowing that bacterial growth doubles every 20 minutes will provide you with an important understanding of safety in this area (Thomson Company, 2005).

Dietary sanitization

The FDA's Food Code defines sanitization as the reduction of bacteria by 5 logs, or 99.999% (Thomson Company, 2005). Therefore, chemical products that are true sanitization agents should be able to reduce bacteria by this amount. This is what differentiates a sanitizer from a cleaning compound. However, the temperature of the water that is being used is also important. Most sanitizing agents have a prescribed water temperature.

Most facilities have three compartment sinks that are used for washing, rinsing, and sanitizing. Again, it is very important to follow the manufacturer's specifications on product use. However, manual sanitizing should abide by the following Food Code guidelines:

- Hot water immersion must be at or higher than 171°F for a minimum of 30 seconds.
- Use of chlorine is typically at 50 parts per million (ppm) at a prescribed water temperature of between 75°F and 100°F.
- Use of iodine is usually between 12.5 and 25 ppm in a water temperature between 75°F and 100°F.
- Quaternary ammonium compounds, often referred to as QUATS, are frequently used in long-term care and often are mixed at 200 ppm. However, it is important to refer to the manufacturer's label before use, as QUATS have a narrow window for toxicity.

Dishwashing machines are common in healthcare facilities due to the sheer volume of residents' trays that must be cleaned. The recommended temperatures for dishwashing machines are as follows (Allen, 2003):

- A minimum of 140°F for washing
- A minimum of 180°F for rinsing

Hazard Analysis Critical Control Points

The Pillsbury Company came up with the process of *Hazard Analysis and Critical Control Points* (HACCP) when it produced foods for NASA astronauts and the space program (Thomson Company, 2005). HACCP is designed to address potential food hazards and issues at particular points during food handling, and is now advocated by the Department of Agriculture and the FDA. The process consists of seven principles.

Principle 1: Analyze hazards

A team approach, hazard analysis brings together individuals who work to identify risks and hazards in the food and dietary handling process. The entire process is analyzed, including contamination, food handling, sanitizing and sterilization techniques, and receipt of food products. Requirements are that the process is a team approach, including people who are familiar with the dietary process and food products, and that it aims to control, minimize, and eliminate any potential hazards.

Principle 2: Identify CCPs

Critical control points (CCPs) are points in the process that can be controlled to eliminate issues that can lead to food hazards. For instance, putting on hairnets in an area outside the kitchen area would be one CCP. Checking dishwasher, refrigerator, and freezer temperatures each day on each shift and assigning a person to oversee that process daily is another CCP.

Principle 3: Establish critical limits

It is important to establish the critical limits for preventive measures associated with the CCPs. To follow this principle, you must determine an appropriate level of acceptability in areas that are controllable, such as freezer and refrigerator temperatures, time periods for holding stock, cooking temperatures, and solutions or chemicals used at appropriate ppm. This is an empirical process that needs to be measured.

Principle 4: Establish procedures to monitor CCPs

This principle highlights the importance of developing a systemic protocol for monitoring the CCPs you've identified. A system needs to be put in place to control the situation and closely monitor for any deviation from acceptable parameters.

Principle 5: Establish corrective action

When parameters for acceptable standards deviate into unacceptable ranges, they need to be acted on immediately. The longer something remains noncompliant, the greater the chance for major problems to occur. The Thomson Company (2005, 100) offers the following as a series of corrective actions:

1. State the problem in an if/then format.

2. Identify the individuals responsible for the corrective action.

3. Determine what the problem is, the corrective action that is needed, and how one can bring the problem back into the appropriate control range.

4. Determine the final dispositions of noncompliant products.

5. Document all actions in writing, with signatures of individuals involved attesting to compliance.

Principle 6: Establish effective recordkeeping

You should document what you did to address and monitor specific issues. It is important not only to keep track of what you did each time you addressed an issue, but also to keep a running log of issues found and how they compare to previous interventions. This is important for trend analysis, which can help you to understand deficiencies and maintain control.

Principle 7: Establish procedures to verify success

You need to verify that the HACCP process is working in an effective manner. The Thomson Company (2005, 101) states that four elements of Principle 7 are important for determining the program's efficacy:

1. Verify that the CCPs are acceptable for establishing control.

2. Ensure that the plan, in its entirety, is sufficiently addressing the issues and maintaining proper control.

3. Reassess the program periodically for its accuracy and efficacy.

4. Ensure that the plan in your facility is functioning in an appropriate manner under appropriate regulatory guidelines.

Handling Linen

Microbial agents can be transferred through improper handling of the linen by the nursing care staff and laundry staff. All too frequently, nursing staff will hold soiled linen too close to their own clothing, thereby infecting their clothing. Then, when they get clean linen, they will hold it the same way, transferring agents that are on their own clothing from the soiled linen onto the clean linen.

This scenario can cause a few major issues. First, the microbial containments that are harbored on the caregiver's uniform are now transferred to clean linen. However, more important, the caregiver has the microbial agents on their person and is carrying them around the healthcare environment, leading to the potential for more widespread microbial outbreaks to occur. This is a major infection containment violation.

Moreover, the healthcare worker is also unnecessarily placing himself or herself at greater risk. No one wants to cultivate a facility of "germphobes," but staff being prudent in their handling of linen may also forestall any unnecessary infections to the workers themselves. This is very important. We frequently become too cavalier in handling linen, especially if there does not seem to be any manifest evidence of blood or other body fluids on the linen. We have to guard against this tendency.

The laundry staff fulfills a very important type of infection control function. However, for these individuals to carry out their laundry duties in an effective manner, they need to be aware of what type of laundry is coming to them. Soiled laundry without blood or body fluids on it may be addressed quite differently than soiled laundry with blood, body fluids or other contaminants on it. Therefore, proper segregation of the linen at the point of disposal needs to be followed: that which is not soiled with blood needs to be identified differently from that which presents more of a biohazard. Therefore, bags that properly inform the workers of what type of linen the bags contain are very necessary for containing infection and for providing protection to the laundry workers who will be receiving the linen. Furthermore, laundry that is clearly marked in different bags provides laundry workers with advanced warning on how to address each type of laundry. Before opening biohazard linen bags, laundry workers will need proper personal protection equipment (PPE), and will also need to know what type of sanitization procedure to use to address the greater level of potential contamination.

As a general rule, soiled linen should be handled as little as possible. Furthermore, moving it around should be avoided to prevent any aerosolization of microbial agents. The soiled laundry hamper should be moved close to the area where soiled linen will be disposed, but not in any resident's room. The amount of distance traveled from the point of linen removal to its disposal should be as short as possible. First, this helps prevent any unnecessary contact with the worker's clothing that may happen when individuals have to walk greater distances. Second, it limits the amount of the facility's environment that is exposed to soiled linen. Having hampers moved close to the room can strongly manage this situation. Before transferring linen to the hamper, it should be bagged and sealed. This is especially important for noticeable biocontaminants that may exist on the linen.

A couple of things need to be monitored to properly contain infection. Soiled linen containers should do just that—contain. Soiled linen containers frequently have compromised or broken lids and fail to adequately contain the soiled linen. Bedspreads and the like are often thrown into these containers without any proper "containment."

Furthermore, soiled linen rooms should have a negative pressure system. This means that the air, along with any microbial agents in it, is moving upward and outward from the soiled utility room and the facility. In fact, the facility should have negative pressure rooms available in the general population area for residents who may have a communicable disease and need to be isolated. Frequently, one can test the negative pressure by placing a piece of paper on the vent and seeing if it is sucked upward and sticks to the vent.

An additional statement should be made about linen that is heavily contaminated by blood, urine, fecal matter, or other types of body fluids. First, no linen should be rinsed off in the resident's room. Linen that is heavily soiled should be immediately placed in a bag, with the bag immediately closed tight, with the exception of those linens that may have fecal matter on it. In this case, remove the fecal matter with a disposable paper towel and dispose of it carefully in the toilet. After that, follow the same procedure. Immediately dispose of the soiled paper towel in a bag that is immediate closed tightly and place it in another biohazard bag for proper identification and disposal. Place the soiled linen in a sealed bag and, then place all linen that is heavily soiled with biocontaminants that go to the laundry in an identifiable biohazard laundry bag or hamper to make the laundry staff aware that this laundry has biocontaminants on it. Make sure that transporting of any biohazard material is done in a manner that prevents any leakage, which could possibly lead to unnecessary environmental contamination in the healthcare facility.

In removing soiled linen, especially that which has noticeable blood, body fluids, or fecal matter on it, make sure that it is always done with gloves and other proper PPEs based on the level of soiled material. This same admonition applies to those in the laundry department. The laundry department is no different than any other area of the healthcare facility and should always have the necessary PPEs available for safe work conditions. Laundry personnel should make sure they are wearing appropriate gloves, aprons, and goggles to avoid the splash risk that may exist in this area, and they should always be highly vigilant about what type of laundry is coming based on laundry coding (i.e., red bags or hampers indicating biohazardous linen). This often entails using a special type of laundry segregation system to identify the different types of washing procedures that are needed for proper sanitization.

Soiled linen should be in 160°F water. When that water temperature is combined with chlorine bleach metered at 50 to 150 parts per million (ppm), it provides significant reduction and removal of most microbial agents from heavily biocontaminated laundry. The Centers for Disease Control (CDC) has stated that studies have shown satisfactory microbial cleansing of soiled linen can be achieved at water temperatures less than 160°F if chemical agents appropriate for lower temperature washing. Always be familiar with the chemical agents used in laundering, and make sure that they are used appropriately and in the required amount stated by the manufacturer. Used at excessive levels, some chemical agents can be toxic.

It is important that laundry or maintenance personnel regularly check water temperature to make sure it meets the required standard for infection control. Temperatures should also be regularly checked in dryers, as well. Washing machines should be regularly inspected to make sure they are moving through their cycles appropriately to completely and thoroughly wash all laundry to proper infection control and safety standards.

Also, laundry staff should be made aware that when they wash loads that may be heavily soiled with biocontaminants, they should thoroughly sanitize the machines, running a non-loaded cycle with proper sanitizing agents before any more laundry is placed into those machines. In most cases, there is usually no further infectious residue left in the machine if proper chemical agents have been used to specification, but at times there may be more resident spores or cysts in the machines that could infect future loads of laundry.

Chapter 4

Policies and Procedures

Introduction

Implementing an infection control program to meet your agency's needs requires a structured process. As a first step, you may want to form a task force to develop, review, and/or revise your facility or organization's policies and procedures.

A policy is best defined as a nonnegotiable directive. It is the rule or mandatory directive that governs the delivery of care by agency staff. For infection control within the long-term care environment, many nonnegotiable directives come from practice acts and from regulations on the federal, state, and local levels. Your agency may designate a particular course of action as one of its own nonnegotiable directives, such as defining time frames. In this chapter, you will find a sample policy that you can modify to fit your agency's needs.

Once a policy is established, it must also delineate how it will be carried out. This is the procedural portion of policy development. Procedures become the map for care delivery. They provide step-by-step guidance for staff. Procedures must reflect your agency's standards and practices as defined in policy while providing the flexibility to allow staff to individualize patient care.

Understanding the differences between policies and procedures is the key to your infection control program's success.

> *Example: The policy statement says the agency implements prevention and control processes including personal hygiene, hand washing and attire, aseptic procedures, personal protective precautions for staff and patients, and cleaning, disinfecting, and/or sterilizing of equipment and supplies. The agency's procedure manual includes those procedures.*

After developing the policies and procedures, follow an organized process for implementation. An emphasis must be placed on "organized." Developing a policy along with its associated procedures needs to follow a logical sequence or it leads to confusion and disarray among the healthcare staff. Furthermore, an organization must establish mechanisms for regular review of the content, policies, and procedures, since new information on infection control, specific diseases, and infection protocol are constantly being updated. Teaching staff and patients' pertinent points must occur through regular in-services, especially if one wants to firmly inculcate these practices into the culture of the organization.

SAMPLE POLICY

> Below is a sample infection control policy. It is meant for purely illustrative purposes. Although it provides a very important structural and procedural example, in reality, one must remember that each infection control policy needs to be tailored to his or her unique healthcare establishment, the clientele served, and the resources available.

PURPOSES

- Describe the scope and requirements of the infection control program.
- Establish a clear sequence of events in the surveillance, identification, reporting, prevention, and control of infection to ensure appropriate services and timely action.
- Ensure compliance with local, state, and federal laws and requirements.
- Ensure that documentation in clinical records, incident reports, and staff health records is accurate and demonstrates appropriate services and action.
- Establish guidelines for staff interaction with patients, families, caregivers, and coworkers that promote appropriate surveillance, prevention, and control of infection.
- Ensure adequate data collection, analysis, assessment, and interpretation of infection findings.
- (Add organization-specific purposes.)

DEFINITIONS

The infection control program is the healthcare facility's program, including policies and procedures, for surveillance, prevention, and control of infection for staff, patients, families, and caregivers. (Add organization-specific definitions.)

POLICY

A. _____ (name of facility or organization) has defined and implemented an infection control program to reduce the risks for infection in residents, families, visitors and healthcare staff.

   1. _____ (name of facility or organization) bases the program on:

      a. Significant infection control issues of the specific patient/resident populations served, including universal (standard) precautions for all patients, caregivers, and staff

      b. Current scientific methods for surveillance and prevention

      c. Epidemiological issues relevant to both residents and staff

      d. Current standards of practice (identify)

      e. Current clinical references (identify); (add others)

   2. _____ (name of facility or organization) coordinates policymaking and planning among all essential components and individuals.

   3. _____ (name of facility or organization) develops protocols to ensure coordination.

B. _____ (name of facility or organization) follows a process to decrease the risk of infection for staff and patients.

   1. _____ (name of facility or organization) ensures that staff comply with:

      a. All infection control policies and procedures

      b. Standard precautions

      c. Universal precautions

2. _____ (name of facility or organization) follows a process to regularly evaluate all products incorporating advances in technology that reduce or eliminate exposure to percutaneous injuries; this process includes:

   a. Product evaluation of medical devices and sharps systems engineered to protect workers before, during, and after use

   b. Input from users of the devices

   c. Documentation of the evaluation process

3. _____ (name of facility or organization) implements the use of safer needle devices whenever possible.

4. _____ (name of facility or organization) requires that staff meet infection control program requirements.

5. The infection control program defines employee health issues.

6. _____ (name of facility or organization) requires staff to follow the Centers for Disease Control and Prevention (CDC) and the Occupational Safety and Health Administration's (OSHA) guidelines for prevention of infection during care delivery.

C. The infection control program includes written policies and procedures related to:

1. Compliance with the documentation and reporting requirements of local, state, and federal rules and regulations, including the CDC, the National Institute for Occupational Safety and Health, (identify others)

2. Placement evaluations (before beginning work), including:

   a. Immunization status or history of vaccine-preventable diseases

   b. History of any conditions that may predispose personnel to acquiring or transmitting infections

   c. Examinations on personnel determined by the health inventory

3. Compliance with accepted professional standards, principles, and practice requirements for employee health and patient care

4. Surveillance systems to track occurrence and transmission of infection, including:

   a. TB screening

   b. Personnel assessments, as required, to evaluate work-related illness or exposures to infectious diseases (identify others)

5. Prevention and control processes, including:

   a. Personal hygiene, hand washing, and attire

   b. Aseptic procedures

   c. Personal protective precautions for staff and patients

   d. Cleaning, disinfecting, and/or sterilizing of equipment and supplies

   e. Supplies intended for single-patient use

   f. Communicable diseases (identify others)

D. _____ (name of facility or organization) ensures staff know and follow infection control policies and procedures by:

1. Providing orientation and annual continuing education programs for staff in prevention and control of infections, including, but not limited to, the following topics:

   a. Bloodborne pathogens exposure—control plan and risk assessment

   b. Personal protective equipment (PPE)

   c. Hand washing and good hygienic practices

   d. Modes of infection transmission

   e. Infection control practices during care delivery

   f. Compliance with standard and universal precautions

   g. Hepatitis B (HBV) vaccination or declination

   h. TB screening

   i. Hazardous materials and waste handling and disposal

   j. Recordkeeping

   k. Exposure incident reporting and investigating

   l. Exposure control plan

   m. Local, state, and federal infection control requirements

   n. Information specific to job responsibilities

   o. Prompt and proper reporting regarding signs and symptoms of infection and disease to supervisory staff

   p. Respiratory protection program and personal respirators as well as proper use and fitting procedures

2. Assessing and documenting staff competencies and proficiencies regarding infection control practices at the time of hire, during orientation, and on a regular basis to be determined by a particular healthcare organization.

3. Providing ongoing staff education and educational resources:

   a. As needed to maintain and improve competence

   b. In content and vocabulary geared toward the educational level, literacy, and language of the employee

E. _____ (name of facility or organization) has a process for identification of infections among residents, families, caregivers, and staff that:

1. Defines types of infections in patients and staff that must be reported (identify)

2. Reviews and analyzes infection data, identifying unusual patterns and trends

3. Reviews patient clinical records for identification of infections, reported and unreported

4. Reviews treatment and services for adequacy and appropriateness of intervention

5. Reviews follow-up on all infection findings to decrease the risk of spreading the infection to other staff, residents, and family members

6. Reviews and reports all nosocomial infections from patients who have been discharged from the hospital or other skilled facilities

7. Reviews and reports all iatrogenic infections that were acquired within your healthcare environment

F. To comply with reporting requirements, _____ (name of facility or organization):

    1. Monitors incidents of infection in staff, patients, and families

    2. Designates an individual to report required infections as defined by the Public Health Service, CDC, or OSHA guidelines

    3. Reports patient or staff illnesses to public health agencies as required by law (usually local and state requirements)

    4. Completes incident reports and infection control logs

    5. Documents any resident's incidents of infection in the clinical records

G. To control infection, _____ (name of facility or organization):

    1. Documents and maintains records of infection occurrences and findings for staff and residents

    2. Provides staff, when ill, with appropriate supplies (such as masks and gloves) or excuses ill staff from resident care or product preparation, if appropriate

    3. Provides education and educational resources on prevention and control of infection for patients, families, and caregivers

    4. Documents resident education in the clinical record

H. _____ (name of facility or organization) addresses job-related illnesses and exposures.

    1. The agency maintains a record of healthcare personnel that includes:

        a. Information obtained during the medical evaluation

        b. Immunization records

        c. Results of tests obtained in any screening or control programs

        d. Reports of work-related illnesses or exposures in accordance with state and federal guidelines

    2. _____ (name of facility or organization) establishes a readily available mechanism for personnel to obtain advice about illnesses they may acquire from or transmit to patients.

    3. _____ (name of facility or organization) evaluates job-related and community-acquired illnesses or important exposures and post-exposure prophylaxis, when indicated.

    4. _____ (name of facility or organization) develops written protocols for handling job-related and community-acquired infectious diseases or significant exposures as required by state and federal guidelines.

    5. Well-developed policies govern:

        a. Personnel responsibility in health service and reporting illness

        b. Removal of personnel from contact with patients/residents and possibly the whole environment

        c. Clearance for work after an infectious disease that required work restriction

    6. _____ (name of facility or organization) identifies persons with authority to relieve personnel of duties.

    7. Work-exclusion policies encourage personnel to report illnesses or exposures and do not penalize them with loss of wages, benefits, or job status.

    8. Latex-sensitivity protocols address:

        a. Evaluation and management of personnel with suspected or known latex allergy

        b. Surveillance for latex reactions

        c. Effectiveness of preventive measures

      d. Identification of patient sensitivities

      e. Staff and patient education issues

      f. Alternative provisions/equipment for workers that have latex sensitivity

I. To meet recordkeeping, data management, and confidentiality requirements, _____ (name of facility or organization):

    1. Maintains updated, confidential records while ensuring appropriate prophylactic management

    2. Maintains confidentiality when releasing data about infections as consistent with HIPAA guidelines

    3. Maintains a personnel database that allows tracking of personnel immunizations, screening tests, and assessments of trends of infections and diseases in personnel

    4. Periodically reviews and assesses data gathered to determine the need for action

    5. Complies with all federal, state, local, and community standards on medical recordkeeping and confidentiality

J. _____ (name of facility or organization)'s quality (performance) improvement activities include infection control to decrease the risk and occurrence of infection through:

    1. Ensuring adequate data collection, analysis, interpretation, and communication of findings

    2. Tracking and trending of infections, including:

      a. Development and implementation of educational programs to address key issues

      b. Implementation of actions to control the incidence of infection

    3. Evaluating the infection control program on a quarterly basis (describe methods)

PROCEDURES

After developing the policy statement, focus your attention on the procedures. Does your agency have all the bases covered? Are there any gaps that you need to fill in? Do the policies and procedures clearly inform staff of your expectations in terms of care delivery? Do they reflect "best practices"? Do your procedures give clear guidance to staff on handling any infection control situations that could occur?

Some "common sense" rules apply to all caregiving situations. Spell out in your infection control policy that staff are not to perform any personal functions, such as eating or drinking, in patient care areas where there is a potential for blood or body fluid exposure. Stress that all procedures should be performed using PPE, if applicable, and in a way that will minimize spraying or splashing of blood and body fluids.

Strong, comprehensive procedures are beneficial when it comes to documentation. If the procedure identifies universal precautions or any other infection control practices, note documentation shows compliance when, for example, staff write, "Performed catheter insertion per procedure."

On the following pages, you'll find samples of more than 20 procedures. These procedures emphasize infection control practices and may not incorporate all care delivery techniques. The language in each procedure serves only as a guide to assist your healthcare organization in developing procedures of its own. You will not be able to use these sample procedures without first analyzing their content.

When developing procedures to carry out policy recommendations, review each procedure's purposes, supplies, and steps. Some procedures specify frequencies, such as "clean the nursing bag once a week." Modify the language of each procedure to fit your healthcare facility's methods. Remember, surveyors will hold you accountable for staff's compliance with procedures. Add procedures as necessary to address all pertinent infection control issues, then educate staff and monitor compliance.

One final element should be added before moving ahead. Keep all procedures clear and well organized. There should always be logical continuity from one step to another, and each step should be as clear and unambiguous as possible. Using the most concise and simple language possible in order to convey all the necessary information in each step is best. Do not attempt to institute terminology that fails to have a clear meaning. As a rule, use language that is easily and unambiguously understood by all.

SAMPLE PROCEDURE

Hand Washing

PURPOSES

- Prevent the transfer of disease-producing organisms from person to person or place to place
- Demonstrate compliance with infection control principles and universal precautions

SUPPLIES

- Liquid soap or Betadine® scrub
- Paper towels
- Nail brush or orange stick
- Plastic trash bag
- Washbasin, pitcher, and bottled water (when no sink or running water is available)
- Approved waterless solution, antiseptic gel, or antiseptic towelette
- Lotion

PROCEDURE

1. Wash hands:
   a. After caring for personal needs, such as using the toilet, blowing nose, covering a sneeze, combing hair, etc.
   b. Before consuming, handling, or serving food or drink
   c. Upon return from public places
   d. Before and after each work shift
   e. Before and after each significant patient contact
   f. Following contact with a contaminated object
   g. After handling waste materials, secretions, drainage, or blood
   h. After handling soiled items, such as linens, clothing, bedpans, urinals, or garbage
   i. Before and after wearing gloves
   j. Before and after touching wounds or performing wound care
   k. After any potential contact with infectious material
2. Procedure for hand washing:
   a. Turn on water and adjust to warm temperature

    b. Rinse hands and lather well with soap and warm water, keeping hands lower than elbows; liquid soap is preferred, as bar soap creates a breeding place for bacteria—if using bar soap, rinse lather from bar soap and return to soap dish

    c. Scrub fingers, palms, backs of hands, wrists, and between fingers for the minimum CDC guidelines of 20 seconds—sing the alphabet or happy birthday song to cover the required time

    d. Clean under fingernails with nail brush or orange stick, if necessary

    e. Rinse hands thoroughly

    f. Use paper towels to dry hands

    g. Use a clean paper towel to turn off faucet

3. Procedure for hand washing when staff cannot leave the bedside (e.g., during a dressing change):

    a. Apply approved waterless solution liberally, or use an antiseptic towelette

    b. Clean the hands for at least 20 seconds, paying attention to fingers, palms, backs of hands, wrists, and spaces between fingers

    c. Dry hands with paper towels

SAMPLE PROCEDURE

Personal Protective Equipment (PPE)

PURPOSES

- Protect patients, family members and friends, and healthcare workers from the spread of infection
- Define circumstances when healthcare workers must wear PPE
- Ensure appropriate use of PPE during patient care delivery
- Demonstrate compliance with infection control principles and universal precautions

SUPPLIES

- Gown (waterproof)
- Goggles or safety eyeglasses with side shields
- Apron (waterproof)
- Face shield
- Gloves
- Personal TB respirator
- Disposable mask
- Hand washing supplies
- Disposable CPR mask
- Alcohol wipes
- Plastic trash bag and a red biohazard trash bag
- 1:10 bleach solution or approved disinfectant for blood/body fluid contamination

PROCEDURE FOR WEARING A GOWN

1. Wear a gown whenever there is the potential for blood or body fluids to splash onto clothes
2. Wash hands
3. Put on the gown; adjust the fit to cover clothing
4. Perform patient care
5. Remove and discard gloves
6. To remove the used gown, grab the inside of the gown (without touching clothing) and roll it into a ball, keeping the contaminated surface inside; avoid touching the outside of the gown
7. If gown is contaminated with visible blood, spray area with a 1:10 bleach solution or approved disinfectant
8. Discard the used gown into a plastic trash bag with the regular garbage
9. Wash hands

PROCEDURE FOR WEARING AN APRON

1. Wear an apron whenever there is the potential for clothing to become contaminated with blood or body fluids by contact with the patient's dressings or linens
2. Wash hands
3. Put on the apron; adjust the fit to cover clothing
4. Perform patient care
5. To remove the soiled apron, grab the garment with gloved hand in front, pull it off, and roll it up with the soiled surface inside
6. If apron is contaminated with visible blood, spray area with a 1:10 bleach solution or approved disinfectant
7. Discard the used apron into a plastic trash bag with the regular garbage
8. Remove and discard gloves
9. Wash hands

PROCEDURE FOR WEARING A FACE MASK

1. Wear a disposable face mask whenever there is a reasonable expectation that blood or other body fluids could be splattered or aerosolized (spread through the air)
2. Make sure the mask is one that has been appropriately fitted to your specifications to make sure there is a proper seal
3. Make sure you apply the face mask appropriately; all individuals should have been trained on appropriate face mask application
4. Wash hands
5. Put on and adjust mask so it covers both the nose and mouth
6. Put on gloves and other PPE as appropriate
7. Perform patient care
8. Change the mask any time it becomes wet
9. Following care delivery, take off and discard the mask:
   a. Using the same gloves if mask is soiled with blood or body fluids
   b. After removing gloves if mask is not soiled with blood or body fluids
10. Remove and discard other PPE according to established procedure
11. Wash hands

PROCEDURE FOR WEARING GOGGLES OR SAFETY EYEGLASSES

1. Wear goggles or safety eyeglasses when there is a reasonable expectation that blood or body fluids might splatter into the eyes

2. Again, make sure that healthcare providers have been fitted with proper googles to their facial contours

3. Make sure healthcare providers have been trained in appropriate use and application of googles

4. Wash hands

5. Apply goggles or glasses and adjust fit; the eye protection should extend from directly over the eyes to all areas around the eyes

6. Put on gloves and other PPE as appropriate

7. Perform patient care

8. Remove the goggles or safety glasses:

    a. Wearing the same gloves if eyewear is soiled with blood or body fluids; set goggles or safety glasses on a barrier for cleaning, if soiled

    b. Remove gloves if eyewear is not soiled with blood or body fluids

9. Remove and discard other PPE according to established procedure

10. Wash hands

11. Wear utility gloves and:

    a. Clean goggles with soap and water after each use

    b. Clean blood-spattered goggles a second time with ethyl alcohol or chlorine compound

    c. Discard cracked or heavily contaminated goggles into a plastic trash bag

12. Wash utility gloves and place them to dry

13. Wash hands

PROCEDURE FOR WEARING A FACE SHIELD

1. Wear a face shield when there is a reasonable expectation that blood or body fluids could be splattered or aerosolized (spread through the air) to the eyes, nose, and mouth

2. Wash hands

3. Apply face shield and adjust fit; again, make sure that the healthcare provider has been properly fitted for a face shield and that they received proper education on how it should be used

4. Apply gloves and other PPE as appropriate

5. Perform patient care

6. Remove the face shield:

    a. Wearing the same gloves, if face shield is soiled with blood or body fluids; set face shield on a barrier for cleaning

    b. After removing gloves if face shield is not soiled with blood or body fluids

7. Remove and discard other PPE according to established procedure

8. Wear utility gloves and:

    a. Clean face shield with soap and water after each use

    b. Clean blood-spattered face shield a second time with ethyl alcohol or chlorine compound

    c. Discard cracked or heavily contaminated face shield in a solid biohazard container to prevent any puncture that can happen if disposed in normal bags

9. Wash utility gloves and place them to dry

10. Wash hands

PROCEDURE FOR WEARING A PERSONAL RESPIRATOR

1. Wear a personal, individually fit-tested respirator whenever making contact with a patient who has active or suspected TB

2. Wash hands

3. Follow the manufacturer's guidelines and protocol for wearing the respirator

4. Perform patient care

5. Wash hands

6. Remove the personal respirator when outside the patient's home; store the respirator in its container

7. Clean hands with antiseptic towelettes; wash hands as soon as possible

8. Follow agency guidelines for regular maintenance and long-term storage

PROCEDURE FOR USING A CARDIOPULMONARY RESUSCITATION (CPR) DEVICE

1. Use a CPR microshield or ventilation device whenever performing CPR

2. Use the device according to manufacturer recommendations

3. Become familiar with the device before its use is required

SAMPLE PROCEDURE

Gloves

PURPOSES

- Protect patients, family members and friends, and healthcare workers from the spread of infection
- Define those circumstances when a healthcare worker should wear gloves
- Define the requirements for use of gloves during patient care delivery
- Demonstrate compliance with infection control principles and universal precautions

SUPPLIES

- Sterile gloves
- Non-sterile gloves
- Utility gloves
- Hand washing supplies
- Plastic trash bag

PROCEDURE

1. Wear gloves whenever there is a reasonable expectation of contact with blood or body fluids

2. Define the use of each type of glove:

    a. Use sterile gloves when working in a sterile field performing any procedure using sterile supplies, such as catheterizations

      b. Use non-sterile gloves when performing personal care if it is likely there will be direct contact with blood or body fluids; examples of such situations include perianal care, handling soiled linens, performing dressing changes not requiring sterile gloves, assisting a patient who is actively bleeding (e.g., from a nosebleed), and examining skin that is abraded or with weeping lesions

      c. Use utility gloves when cleaning equipment, the work area, or spills, and when doing housekeeping chores that involve potential exposure to blood and body fluids

3. To apply sterile gloves:

      a. Remove any jewelry that could puncture the gloves

      b. Wash hands and dry thoroughly

      c. Set the package containing the sterile gloves on a clean surface (e.g., on clean paper towels)

      d. Open the package carefully, peeling the outward, non-sterile covering away from the inside, sterile portion of the package

      e. Using your nondominant hand, grasp the sterile glove at the top by its inside cuff; do not touch the outside of the glove

      f. Slide dominant hand into the sterile glove

      g. Pick up the other glove by sliding the sterile gloved fingers under the inside cuff, without touching the exposed hand

      h. Adjust the fit, using fingers as necessary

      i. Avoid touching anything outside of the sterile field while wearing sterile gloves

      j. Remove the gloves if at any time they become soiled or contaminated, wash hands, and begin again with a new pair

4. To apply non-sterile gloves:

      a. Remove any jewelry that could puncture the gloves

      b. Wash hands and dry thoroughly

      c. Put on the gloves carefully, taking care not to tear or puncture them

5. To remove both sterile and non-sterile gloves:

      a. Grasp the cuff of one glove with the opposite gloved hand

      b. Pull the glove downward carefully, turning it inside out as it is removed, and crunch it into a ball in the gloved hand

      c. Continue holding the removed glove with the gloved hand

      d. Grasp the inside top of the cuff of the gloved hand with the ungloved hand (this is considered to be the cleanest part of the glove)

      e. Peel the glove downward carefully, turning it inside out over the other glove

      f. Discard both gloves in a plastic trash bag immediately; for surgical gloves and nonsurgical gloves that have come into contact with body fluids, wounds, or possible infectious contaminant, dispose within labeled biohazard trash bags

      g. Wash hands

      h. Never wash or try to decontaminate disposable gloves

6. To use utility gloves:

      a. Wash hands and dry thoroughly

      b. Put on the gloves

c. Inspect the gloves for cracking, peeling, or tearing

d. Clean undamaged gloves with detergent and hot water

e. Remove and place the gloves on a clean surface to dry

f. Dispose of gloves with any tears or cracks

SAMPLE PROCEDURE

Latex Sensitivity

PURPOSE
- Define a protocol for those staff and patients who develop or present with an allergy to latex gloves or medical equipment containing latex

SUPPLIES
- Non-latex substitute products

PROCEDURE
1. Educate staff on latex allergy, its signs and symptoms, and risk groups
2. Identify latex products
3. Define a reporting mechanism and a protocol for cases of latex sensitivity
4. Identify replacement products to protect the allergic party from exacerbation of an existing allergic condition
5. Eliminate the use of latex gloves, whenever possible, in homes where patients or staff experience latex sensitivity
6. Track the incidence and handling of latex sensitivity cases

SAMPLE PROCEDURE

Blood Specimen Collection

Although most blood specimen collections are done by lab technicians/phlebotomists, who are contracted by the nursing care facility, there are times when specimens may be drawn by qualified long-term care staff.

PURPOSES
- Ensure proper collection, labeling, and handling of specimens
- Demonstrate compliance with infection control principles and universal precautions
- Make sure that it is only completed by those trained and/or certified to carry out these procedures

SUPPLIES
- Tourniquet
- Barrier
- Alcohol wipes
- Specimen container
- Syringe
- Needles (18 and 22 gauge)

- Label
- Blood specimen tubes—specific to the type of collection
- Transportation container or plastic lab biohazard specimen bag
- Gloves
- Hand washing supplies
- Bandages, gauze, tape
- Arm board

PROCEDURE

1. Verify the physician's order for specimen collection
2. Confirm that the patient has observed the proper procedure for preparation
3. Prepare supplies and label the specimen container
4. Explain the procedure and prepare the patient
5. Wash hands and dry thoroughly
6. Apply gloves
7. Collect the specimen in the labeled tube
8. Discard the syringe and needle in one piece into a sharps container
9. Provide any post-collection care to the patient (if gloves are soiled with blood, remove and wash hands before assisting the patient, and put on another pair of gloves, if necessary)
10. Place the specimen tube(s) in a sealed, puncture-resistant, biohazard-labeled container for transport to the laboratory
11. Remove and discard gloves, and wash hands
12. Document collection of the specimen, noting the time, date, and type of specimen, any pertinent patient comments or observations, and destination
13. Transport the specimen as assigned

SAMPLE PROCEDURE

Urine Specimen Collection

PURPOSES

- Ensure proper collection, labeling, and handling of specimens
- Demonstrate compliance with infection control principles and universal precautions

SUPPLIES

Depending on the patient's voiding ability as well as type of specimen (clean catch or not) supplies may include:

- Specimen container
- Label
- Antiseptic cleansing solution
- Sealable, leak-proof biohazard bag
- Hemostat (clamp)

- Gloves (sterile or non-sterile)
- Urinal or specimen "hat" or cup
- Disposable catheter set
- Hand washing supplies
- Leak-proof pad
- Alcohol prep pad
- Sterile needle and syringe (if applicable)

PROCEDURE

1. Verify the physician's order for specimen collection
2. Explain the procedure to the resident if they are able to understand
3. Some samples may need to be collected from resident by healthcare staff, especially when resident needs assistance to stand, ambulate, etc.
4. Position the patient or assist to the bathroom or commode
5. Prepare supplies and label the specimen container
6. Wash hands and dry thoroughly
7. Apply gloves
8. Put on a gown, apron, mask, and/or goggles if there is the possibility of splashing
9. For the patient with an indwelling catheter, cleanse the aspiration port with an alcohol wipe to avoid cross-contamination of microorganisms into the tubing
10. If performing a catheterization, follow established procedure
11. Collect the specimen in the labeled container
12. Provide any post-collection care to the patient (if gloves are soiled with blood or body fluids, remove and wash hands before assisting patient, and put on another pair of gloves)
13. Place the specimen cup in a sealed biohazard-labeled bag for transport to the laboratory
14. Remove and discard gloves and personal protective equipment, and wash hands
15. Document collection of the specimen, noting the time, date, and type of specimen, any pertinent patient comments or observations, and destination
16. Transport the specimen as assigned or instruct the patient how to store it safely until pickup

SAMPLE PROCEDURE

Stool Specimen Collection

PURPOSES

- Ensure proper collection, labeling, and handling of specimens
- Demonstrate compliance with infection control principles and universal precautions

SUPPLIES

- Specimen cup or slide
- Gloves
- Sealable, leak-proof biohazard bag

- Bedpan
- Label
- Specimen collection "hat"
- Tongue blades
- Hand washing supplies
- Paper towels

PROCEDURE

1. Verify the physician's order for specimen collection
2. Prepare supplies and label the specimen container
3. Position the patient or assist to the bathroom or commode
4. Wash hands and dry thoroughly
5. Apply non-sterile gloves
6. Put on a gown, apron, mask, and/or goggles if there is the possibility of splashing
7. Collect the specimen in the labeled container
8. Provide any post-collection care to the patient (if gloves are soiled with blood or body fluids, remove and wash hands before assisting patient, and put on another pair of gloves)
9. Place the specimen cup in a sealed biohazard-labeled bag for transport to the laboratory
10. Remove and discard gloves and personal protective equipment, and wash hands
11. Document collection of the specimen, noting the time, date, and type of specimen, any pertinent patient comments or observations, and destination
12. Transport the specimen as assigned

SAMPLE PROCEDURE

Sputum Specimen Collection

PURPOSES
- Ensure proper collection, labeling, and handling of specimens
- Demonstrate compliance with infection control principles and universal precautions

SUPPLIES
Supplies will depend on whether the specimen is expectorated or suctioned, but may include:
- Sterile specimen container
- Tissues
- Sealable, leak-proof biohazard bag
- Lubricant
- Label
- Normal saline
- Gloves
- Hand washing supplies

- Emesis basin
- Suction equipment with in-line specimen container

PROCEDURE

1. Verify the physician's order for specimen collection.

2. Explain to the resident, if they are able to understand, the reason and need for the specimen

3. Explain the procedure to the patient

4. Prepare supplies and label the specimen container

5. Position the patient

6. Wash hands and dry thoroughly

7. Put on a mask, goggles, and/or face shield if the patient must cough forcefully or if the specimen is being obtained while suctioning the trachea

8. Wear gloves while collecting the specimen; wear sterile gloves if obtaining the specimen by suctioning the tracheostomy

9. Following suctioning, disconnect the catheter from the in-line trap and gather it up using the dominant hand; pull the glove cuff inside out and down around the used catheter to seal it for disposal

10. If the specimen was collected by the patient, wipe the exterior of the container with alcohol to prevent cross-contamination

11. Provide any post-collection care to the patient (if gloves are soiled with blood or body fluids, remove and wash hands before assisting patient, and put on another pair of gloves)

12. Place the specimen cup in a sealed biohazard-labeled bag for transport to the laboratory

13. Remove and discard gloves and personal protective equipment, and wash hands

14. Document collection of the specimen, noting the time, date, and type of specimen, any pertinent patient comments or observations, and destination

15. Transport the specimen as assigned

SAMPLE PROCEDURE

Infection Control Practices During Wound Care and Dressing Changes

PURPOSES

- Prevent the spread of infectious diseases
- Demonstrate compliance with infection control principles and universal precautions
- Ensure proper handling, labeling, and disposal of all contaminated dressings according to local, state, and federal regulations

SUPPLIES

- Gloves (non-sterile and/or sterile)
- Clean dressing (as ordered)
- Tape (adhesive or paper) or appropriate supplies used to secure dressing
- Scissors (if using adhesive tape to secure dressing)
- Topical treatment (as ordered)

- Solution for irrigation (as ordered)
- Hand washing supplies, including antiseptic gel or waterless soap
- Plastic trash bag
- 1:10 bleach solution or approved disinfectant

PROCEDURE

1. Verify the physician's order for wound care
2. Gather all the supplies required for the dressing change, such as dressings, tape, scissors, specific treatment items, and a disposal bag, and place them in a clean area near the patient; make sure there is a clean field to prevent touching of sterile material with non-sterile or fomitic elements
3. Explain the procedure to the patient
4. Position the patient, ensuring privacy and comfort
5. Wash hands and dry thoroughly
6. Put on an apron or gown
7. Apply non-sterile or sterile gloves based on the invasive nature of the wound and the potential for secondary infection
8. Remove the present dressings by lifting gently, touching only the top part of the clean corner
    a. Remove existing tape carefully to protect skin integrity
    b. Handle the dressing carefully
    c. Observe for signs of drainage
    d. Discard the contaminated dressing in a disposal bag and subsequently into a biohazard bag; assess/observe the wound
9. Remove and discard gloves, and wash hands (if unable to leave the patient to wash hands, use waterless soap or antiseptic gel)
10. Unwrap the new dressing carefully
11. Apply a new pair of sterile or non-sterile gloves, as determined by the procedure
12. Perform the wound care procedure according to the plan of care, following established procedures
13. Apply the clean dressing directly to the wound; limit taping on fragile skin
14. Remove gloves and any personal protective equipment following established procedure and discard
15. Wash hands again
16. Report and document evidence of foul odor, bleeding, increased drainage, or changes in the appearance of the wound, drainage, or temperature of the skin
17. Document the procedure
18. Disinfect any surfaces soiled with blood or drainage using a 1:10 bleach solution or approved disinfectant, including any whirlpool or other wound care equipment

SAMPLE PROCEDURE

Infection Control Practices During Daily Personal Care

PURPOSES

- Prevent the spread of infectious diseases
- Demonstrate compliance with infection control principles and universal precautions

SUPPLIES

- Non-sterile gloves
- Soap
- Toothbrush
- Water
- Toothpaste
- Towels
- Shampoo
- Washcloths
- Brush, comb
- Hand washing supplies
- Incontinence products
- Razor/electric shaver
- Patient-specific toiletries, lotions, powders, deodorants, etc.

PROCEDURE FOR BATHING

1. Verify the assignment for bathing
2. Gather all the supplies and place them in a clean area near the patient
3. Explain the procedure to the patient
4. Position the patient, ensuring privacy and comfort
5. Wash hands and dry thoroughly
6. Apply non-sterile gloves if the patient's skin is broken or bleeding and/or to bathe the perineal area
7. Apply other PPE as appropriate for the situation
8. Bathe the patient or assist with bathing as appropriate
   a. Work from cleaner to dirtier areas
   b. Change water, gloves, and supplies as indicated when moving from a dirtier to a cleaner area
9. Assist with or dry the patient thoroughly—pat dry to prevent skin tears
10. Apply any after-bath products (e.g., lotions, powders, or deodorant) as appropriate
11. Remove and discard gloves and PPE, when appropriate, following established procedure
12. Dress the patient in appropriate attire
13. Wash hands
14. Document the bath and pertinent observations

PROCEDURE FOR PERFORMING PERINEAL CARE FOR THE FEMALE RESIDENT

1. Verify the assignment

2. Gather all the supplies and place them in a clean area near the resident

3. Explain the procedure to the resident and make sure approval is given

4. Position the resident, ensuring privacy and comfort; drape a bath blanket over the patient

5. Wash hands and dry thoroughly

6. Apply non-sterile gloves

7. Apply other PPE as appropriate for the situation

8. Use a minimum of soap and a soft washcloth, working from cleaner to dirtier areas

9. Carefully wash the skin folds formed by the inner thigh and outer labia, working from the pubic area to the rectum and avoiding contact with anal area

10. Separate the folds of the labia with one hand and, using downward strokes, wash very gently; use a different section of the washcloth for each stroke

11. Rinse thoroughly and pat dry

12. Help patient turn onto side

13. To remove any fecal material:
    a. Wipe the anal area with toilet tissue, using one backward stroke
    b. Start at the posterior vaginal area and wipe from front to back
    c. Properly dispose of tissue

14. Use a clean washcloth to wash and rinse area

15. Dry area gently but thoroughly

16. Apply any topical medications as assigned or a thin layer of powder, if desired

17. Observe skin condition

18. Apply a clean incontinence product as appropriate

19. Clean and put away equipment; remove gloves and discard when appropriate

20. Wash hands and dry thoroughly

21. Document care delivery and any observations

PROCEDURE FOR PERFORMING PERINEAL CARE FOR THE MALE RESIDENT

1. Verify the assignment

2. Gather all the supplies and place them in a clean area near the resident

3. Explain the procedure to the resident and make sure approval is provided

4. Position the patient, ensuring privacy and comfort; drape a bath blanket over the resident Wash hands and dry thoroughly

5. Apply non-sterile gloves

6. Apply other PPE as appropriate for the situation

7. Use a minimum of soap and a soft washcloth, working from cleaner to dirtier areas

8. Hold shaft of penis with one hand; move washcloth from tip down, toward pubic area
    a. Clean tip of penis
    b. Using a circular motion, start at urethral opening and work outward with a washcloth or cotton ball

    c. If resident is uncircumcised, gently retract foreskin when cleaning

    d. Rinse area with a clean washcloth or cotton ball

9.   Wash scrotum and surrounding skin folds

10.   Rinse thoroughly and pat dry

11.   Help patient turn onto side

12.   To remove any fecal material:

    a. Wipe the anal area with toilet tissue, using one backward stroke

    b. Start at the posterior scrotal area and wipe from front to back

    c. Properly dispose of tissue

13.   Use a clean washcloth to wash and rinse area

14.   Dry area gently but thoroughly

15.   Apply any topical medications as assigned or a thin layer of powder, if desired

16.   Observe skin condition

17.   Apply a clean incontinence product as appropriate

18.   Clean and put away equipment; remove and discard gloves when appropriate

19.   Wash hands and dry thoroughly

20.   Document care delivery and any observations

PROCEDURE FOR PERFORMING HAIR CARE

1.   Verify the assignment

2.   Gather all the supplies and place them in a clean area near the patient

3.   Explain the procedure to the resident and obtain approval

4.   Position the patient, ensuring privacy and comfort

5.   Wash hands and dry thoroughly

6.   Apply non-sterile gloves if the patient's scalp contains sores, broken skin, or lice

7.   Assist or wash the patient's hair and scalp thoroughly, following established procedure

8.   Dry the patient's scalp and hair with a towel

9.   Assist with, or comb or brush the patient's hair; blow dry if preferred

10.   Clean and put away equipment; remove and discard gloves when appropriate

11.   Wash hands and dry thoroughly

12.   Document care delivery and any observations

PROCEDURE FOR PERFORMING MOUTH CARE

1.   Verify the assignment

2.   Gather all the supplies and place them in a clean area near the patient

3.   Explain the procedure to the resident and obtain resident's approval

4.   Wash hands and dry thoroughly

5.   Apply non-sterile gloves

6.   Assist with or perform mouth care following established procedure

7. Remove and discard gloves

8. Wash hands and dry thoroughly

9. Document care delivery and any observations

SAMPLE PROCEDURE

Handling Waste and Disposables

PURPOSES

- Prevent the spread of infectious diseases

- Ensure proper handling, labeling, and disposal of all wastes according to local, state, and federal regulations

- Demonstrate compliance with infection control principles and universal precautions

SUPPLIES

- A commercial sharps container that is puncture proof, red, labeled with a biohazard sign, and leak-proof plastic trash bag with biohazard identification

- Trash container

- Non-sterile gloves

- 1:10 bleach solution or agency-approved disinfectant

- Hand washing supplies

PROCEDURE FOR DISPOSAL OF SHARPS

1. Wash hands and apply gloves as appropriate

2. Administer injection or perform procedure according to the plan of care and following established procedures

3. Handle the syringe or sharp carefully to avoid injury—do not recap!

4. Dispose of used syringes and sharps immediately following injection or procedure; never recap the syringe or break off the needle

5. Remove and discard gloves and wash hands when appropriate

6. Never manually open, empty, or clean a reusable, contaminated sharps disposal container

7. Check the sharps container periodically to make sure there is still enough room to dispose of whole syringes and attached needles; a good rule of thumb is never to fill the container more than two-thirds full to allow adequate space

8. When the sharps container is full:

   a. Seal the sharps container securely

   b. Follow facility policy for disposal of biohazard material with appropriate contracted disposal agency

PROCEDURE FOR DISPOSAL OF USED IV BAGS, TUBING, FOLEY BAGS, SUCTION CANISTERS, ETC.

1. Wash hands and apply non-sterile gloves

2. Empty all fluid from IV bags and tubing before discarding in biohazard trash; discard all needles into a sharps container; drain and rinse body waste containers, such as Foley bags, suction canisters, and their tubing, before placing in the biohazard trash

3. Place emptied tubing, drainage bags, or canisters in a plastic bag and place in the trash

4. Secure trash and place in designated area for pickup with appropriately identified biohazard bag markings

5. Remove and discard gloves

6. Wash hands

PROCEDURE FOR DISPOSAL OF PATIENT WASTE

1. Wash hands and apply non-sterile gloves

2. Pour patient feces, urine, blood, and emesis into the toilet carefully, to avoid splashing

3. Flush the toilet

4. Clean emesis container, bedpan, urinal, or toilet with soap and hot water

5. Remove and discard gloves

6. Wash hands

PROCEDURE FOR DISPOSAL OF BANDAGES, DRESSINGS, CATHETERS, GLOVES, INCONTINENCE PADS, AND DRAINAGE RECEPTACLES

1. Wash hands and apply non-sterile gloves

2. Perform removal of bandages, dressings, catheters, incontinence pads, or drainage receptacles

3. Spray or pour a 1:10 bleach solution or approved disinfectant on dressings that are soiled with blood or body fluid before placing in a plastic trash bag for disposal

4. Wrap dressings soiled with blood or body fluid in a plastic bag, tie the bag, and dispose of this bag in marked biohazard bag or container; double bag articles soiled with blood or body fluid if they are heavily contaminated and there is the potential for leakage; discard them in the biohazard marked garbage

5. Remove and discard gloves; wash hands

6. Tie the plastic trash bag securely and dispose of it according to local laws; never push down on trash in the bag when attempting to tie the bag for disposal, as the bag could contain sharps or other harmful material

7. Wash hands

SAMPLE PROCEDURE

Environmental Practices

PURPOSES

- Prevent the growth of microorganisms
- Prevent the spread of infection
- Maintain a clean environment
- Maintain clean equipment
- Demonstrate compliance with infection control principles and universal precautions

SUPPLIES

- Disinfectant/disinfectant spray (specifically advertised as effective in HIV decontamination)
- Paper towels
- Plastic trash bag
- 1:10 bleach solution
- Detergent or soap
- White vinegar and water (1:3)
- Hand washing supplies
- 70% isopropyl alcohol
- Alcohol wipes
- 3% hydrogen peroxide
- Lysol broom
- Other commercial products effective for decontamination approved by CDC and OSHA guidelines
- Dustpan
- Non-sterile or utility gloves

PROCEDURE TO CLEAN UP BLOOD AND BODY FLUID SPILLS

1. Wash hands and apply gloves
2. Carefully wipe up spill with paper towels
3. Discard the paper towels in a plastic trash bag, taking care not to contaminate the outside of the bag
4. Spray with disinfectant or bleach spray until area is glistening wet
5. Allow area to dry; keep people and pets out of the area until completely dry
6. Remove and discard gloves
7. Wash hands

PROCEDURE FOR CLEANING EQUIPMENT

1. Follow the facility/organization schedule and procedure for cleaning stethoscopes, baby scales, glucose monitors, thermometers, hemostats, clamps, physical therapy equipment, respiratory therapy equipment, speech-language pathology equipment, commodes, bedpans, urinals, and other equipment
2. Choose the appropriate disinfectant for the item and follow directions carefully

3. Wear utility gloves when using commercial disinfectants and bleach; wear goggles if the solution is highly caustic and could splash into the eyes; choose an area that is well ventilated

4. Wash items with soap and water first, then use a disinfectant; submerge the item, when possible, for the directed amount of time to get the best results; dry thoroughly

5. Discard items used to disinfect equipment in a leak-proof plastic bag (discard disposable gloves along with items used to disinfect the equipment; if utility gloves were used, wash with soap and water, then place them in an area to dry that is removed from contact with other health workers and residents; secure the plastic bag and dispose in an identifiable biohazard bag or container; follow state and local infectious material disposal regulations)

6. Wash hands

KITCHEN AND FOOD HANDLING GUIDELINES

- Wash hands
- Clean the tops of cans before opening them
- Wash fruits and vegetables before serving
- Cook all types of meat, fish, and eggs thoroughly
- Refrigerate perishable foods
- Never eat or serve spoiled food
- Wash dishes, including those used by the patient, in hot soapy water or using the hot cycle of the dishwasher; the machine wash cycle should be as follows:
    —A minimum of 140°F for washing
    —A minimum of 180°F for rinsing
- Wipe cooking and eating surfaces regularly
- Mop floors weekly and as needed
- Wrap and remove garbage daily
- Make sure food is refrigerated at or under 40°F
- Make sure the freezer temperature is at or below 0°F
- Make sure all foods are stored a minimum of 6 inches above floor level
- Make sure food is cooked thoroughly

BATHROOM CLEANING GUIDELINES

- Wash hands and apply gloves as appropriate
- Flush the toilet after each use
- Make sure there are disposable paper hand towels
- Clean toilet/restroom area daily
- Mop the floor at least once a week

SAMPLE PROCEDURE

Handling Linens

PURPOSES

- Prevent the spread of infection when changing linens soiled with blood or body fluids

- Promote a clean environment

- Demonstrate compliance with infection control principles and universal precautions

SUPPLIES

- Gloves (non-sterile or utility)

- Pillowcase, laundry bag, or plastic bag

- Washing machine

- Detergent

- Bleach

- Clean linen

- Hand washing supplies

PROCEDURE FOR CHANGING LINENS SOILED WITH BLOOD OR BODY FLUIDS

1. Wash hands

2. Survey the room and identify a place to set both the soiled and clean linen; set the clean linen on the seat of a chair or a bedside table if washed, or clean before use

3. Apply non-sterile or utility gloves and apron

4. Loosen linens on bed carefully, continuously watching for items that could be hidden in the bedclothes; avoid shaking or fanning linens

5. Remove soiled linens carefully, folding the cleaner portion over the stained area
   a. Those without body fluid containments are placed in a separate type of bag to notify laundry personnel that these are not biohazard risks
   b. Those that have infectious elements or body fluids on them should be clearly sent to laundry within an appropriately marked bag that indicates biohazard risk and special procedures to be employed by laundry personnel

6. Put the soiled linens in a plastic bag or plastic-lined container, to avoid leakage of contaminated contents
   a. Take care not to let soiled linens touch clothing
   b. Carry linens away from the body
   c. Never place linens on the floor

7. Wash soiled linens as soon as possible to avoid the growth and spread of bacteria

8. Remove and discard gloves

9. Wash hands

10. Complete linen change:
    a. Open and spread clean linen on the bed
    b. Observe principles of asepsis
    c. Avoid shaking or fanning linens

PROCEDURE FOR LAUNDERING LINENS SOILED WITH BLOOD OR BODY FLUIDS

1. Wash hands

2. Apply gloves

3. Presoak linens soiled with blood or body fluids in cold water

   a. Use detergent plus one cup of bleach, as appropriate; use the manufacturers' specification for using specific chemical products that are used to address biohazard decontamination—some of the products have narrow windows of toxicity

   b. Set on the hottest cycle available for at least 25 minutes

   c. Run the wash cycle twice, if necessary, to wash for an adequate amount of time

4. Remove gloves and wash hands

5. Dry laundry on regular setting

6. Disinfect a contaminated washing machine by running an empty cycle, using either a commercial disinfectant or one cup of full-strength bleach

7. Discuss with the supervisor what to do in situations when there is no washing machine, dryer, or running water

SAMPLE PROCEDURE

Blood and Body Fluids Exposure Incident

PURPOSES

- Take effective, immediate action to reduce contamination or injury after an exposure incident

- Take protective measures to reduce the effects of contamination

- Promote complete and proper documentation of the incident

- Demonstrate compliance with infection control principles and universal precautions

SUPPLIES

- Water (bottled if fresh water is unavailable)

- Soap

- Antiseptic

- First aid kit

PROCEDURE FOR EXPOSURE TO BLOOD AND BODY FLUIDS

1. Define an exposure incident (an exposure incident occurs any time a person comes in contact with blood or potentially infectious body fluid that can enter the bloodstream through chapped or broken skin, open wounds, mucous membranes, or a needlestick)

2. Clean any area exposed to the patient's blood or body fluid immediately, as the exposure can lead to an infection by bloodborne pathogens

   a. Irrigate exposed eyes or other mucous membranes with clean water, saline solution, or sterile irrigation solution for at least five minutes; make sure irrigation sites are readily available in all nursing areas for quick and immediate access

    b. Wash any exposed area, especially open cuts or sores, with soap and water. Use of caustic agents, such as bleach, is not recommended

    c. Wash the area with soap and water; apply antiseptic

    d. Carefully save any sharps or items involved for testing; transport separately in a sharps container

    e. Wash any body part exposed to infectious material vigorously with soap and water

    f. Change clothing immediately if soiled with blood or body fluids; wash the contaminated articles in a 1:10 bleach solution

3. Notify the clinical supervisor immediately to report the exposure incident and obtain follow-up instructions

    a. Prompt reporting is essential because, in some cases, HIV post-exposure treatment may be recommended; this treatment should be started as soon as possible, preferably within one to two hours following exposure

    b. The supervisor must notify the agency's infection control manager within 12 hours of the exposure

4. Complete and submit an exposure incident report to the infection control manager within 24 hours of the exposure; also complete the necessary OSHA incident forms for worker exposure and incidents

    a. Document the entire incident and include the path of exposure

    b. Identify the name of the infected source, unless prohibited by state or local law

PROCEDURE FOR FOLLOW-UP ON EXPOSURE TO BLOOD AND BODY FLUIDS

1. If at all possible, obtain consent from the resident who led to the worker's exposure and test the source blood as soon as possible to identify the pathogen, unless the source is already known to be either HBV and/or HIV positive; notify the patient's physician of incident

    a. Document the reason if the source refuses to grant consent for blood work

    b. The facility must reveal the source test results to the exposed employee, along with disclosure laws and regulations regarding the infected source's right to confidentiality

    c. Most states have laws that allow for patients to be tested even if they refuse consent due to the public health factor involved

2. Collect and test the exposed employee's blood for HBV and HIV status

    a. Obtain consent for testing; the employee has up to 90 days following exposure to consent, and has the right to decline

    b. If the employee allows baseline collection but refuses HIV analysis, keep the collected blood sample for a minimum of 90 days; if the employee changes his or her mind during that time, analyze the collected sample as soon as possible

    c. Document accordingly

3. Introduce appropriate post-exposure prophylaxis

    a. Inform the exposed employee about the recommended follow-up based on current knowledge of epidemiology, the risk (if known) of transmitting the infection to others, and the methods of preventing transmission to others

    b. Inform the exposed employee about the options for prophylaxis, the risk (if known) of infection when treatment is not accepted, the degree of protection afforded by the therapy, and the potential side effects

4. Schedule an appointment with a healthcare professional for medical evaluation of the employee as soon as possible following exposure

5. Obtain and provide the employee with a copy of the healthcare professional's written opinion within 15 days of medical evaluation

   a. The communication must include evidence that the employee received information regarding the results of the examination and any medical conditions that require further treatment

   b. All other findings or diagnoses should remain confidential and are not to be included in the written report

   c. Managers are not privileged to this information

6. Report the exposure incident on the OSHA 300 Series form if:

   a. Medical treatment beyond first aid is required

   b. The incident results in seroconversion

   c. The incident is work-related and involves loss of consciousness, transfer to a healthcare facility, and/or restricted duties

7. Counsel the employee as appropriate

8. Evaluate reported illnesses as appropriate

9. Investigate the circumstances surrounding the incident to evaluate whether additional prevention strategies need to be implemented

Form 4.1: Blood and body fluids exposure incident report

Name: _____

Address: _____

Ph#: _____ Position: _____

Incident date:_____ Time: _____ AM PM

Date reported: _____ Time: _____ AM PM

Reported to:_____ Date:_____ Time: _____ AM PM

Where exposure occurred:

❑ Patient home

❑ Outside home

Witnesses:

❑ No

❑ Yes

Name:_____

Ph#: _____

PPE used at time of exposure:

❑ Gloves   ❑ Mask

❑ Gown   ❑ Goggles/eye shield

❑ Apron   ❑ Other:_____

❑ None (Why? _____)

❑ Sharp puncture/needlestick

Type: _____

Purpose: _____

Contaminated: ❑ Yes   ❑ No   ❑ Unknown

Location: _____

Depth of injury: _____

   Superficial: _____ Moderate: _____ Deep: _____

Mucous membrane exposure: ❑ Yes   ❑ No   Amt:_____

Exposed body part:

❑ Intact skin

❑ Non-intact skin

❑ Eyes   ❑ Nose

❑ Mouth   ❑ Other:

Body fluids involved:

❑ Blood or blood products   ❑ Urine   ❑ Feces

❑ Drainage: Type   ❑ Vomit   ❑ Sputum

❑ Visibly contaminated solution (water used to clean spill)

Source: Resident knows: ❑ Yes   ❑ No   ❑ Unknown

Describe how the exposure occurred and the job duties that were being performed: _____

_____

Describe immediate postexposure treatment: _____

_____

Date: _____ Time: _____ AM PM

Follow-up treatment:

❑ Refused   ❑ Physician: _____

❑ No treatment   ❑ Emergency room: _____ ❑ Other_____

❑ Employee HBV vaccine   Date: _____

Employee signature: _____ Date: _____

Administrative comments: _____

Administrative signature:_____ Date: _____

SAMPLE PROCEDURE

Blood and Body Fluids Exposure Control Plan

PURPOSES

- Document procedures used in controlling exposure to bloodborne or airborne pathogens
- Define and communicate procedures for staff to follow when exposed to pathogens including, but not limited to, HIV, hepatitis, and other bloodborne pathogens from needlesticks or splashes of blood or body fluids that come in contact with open skin or mucous membranes
- Demonstrate compliance with OSHA regulations regarding follow-up testing, counseling, and post-exposure treatment

SUPPLIES

- Binder containing exposure control plan
- Training program materials
- Forms

PROCEDURE

1. Identify:

    a. Those job classifications where there is potential risk for occupational exposure to bloodborne pathogens.

    b. Tasks and procedures within each job classification that involve exposure risk

    c. Highly hazardous procedures

    d. Policies and protocols for early detection and treatment for staff exposure

2. Describe ways to minimize exposure:

    a. Communicate hazardous situations to staff ahead of time, when possible

    b. Define and communicate the types of personal protective equipment required for all the different kinds of potential infectious opportunities for each patient

3. Teach staff in annual mandatory in-service about:

    a. Preventive measures in place, such as vaccine protocols for HBV

    b. The continuous use of universal precautions

    c. Measures to minimize the risk of exposure

4. Provide instructions on what to do immediately following an exposure to minimize the possibility of becoming infected:

    a. Take appropriate actions

    b. Provide the name and number of whom to contact should any exposure occur

    c. Explain how important it is to contact the designated individual at the overseeing infection control within your healthcare facility/organization immediately following any exposure incident; in some cases, HIV post-exposure treatment may be recommended, and this treatment should be started as soon as possible, preferably within one to two hours following exposure

    d. Provide instruction on what to do should the exposure occur during on-call hours

5. Assess and treat all exposure incidents

6. Ensure documentation of the incident:

   a. Teach staff about an incident report, where they are kept, how and when to fill them out, and to whom these forms should be submitted

   b. The supervisor must notify the agency's infection control manager within 12 hours of the exposure

   c. Employees who suffer exposure to any infectious disease cannot care for patients until cleared by the infection control manager

7. Provide post-exposure testing and treatment, including counseling, according to Public Health Service, CDC, and OSHA guidelines

8. Maintain confidentiality

9. Report on the OSHA 300 form any exposure incident:

   a. If medical treatment beyond first aid is required

   b. That results in seroconversion

   c. That is work-related and involves loss of consciousness, transfer, and/or restricted duties

10. Establish procedures for evaluating the circumstances surrounding each exposure incident for purposes of quality (performance) improvement

11. Store the plan where staff can easily access and review it

12. Evaluate and update the plan annually and any time a policy or procedure changes that directly or indirectly affects the original plan

SAMPLE PROCEDURE

Hepatitis B (HBV) Vaccine

PURPOSES
- Provide staff with patient contact protection from exposure to HBV
- Comply with the OSHA's Bloodborne Pathogens standard

SUPPLIES
- Employee information sheet
- HBV vaccine log
- Consent/declination form
- HBV vaccine (with manufacturer's package insert)
- Alcohol wipe
- Disposable syringe
- Non-sterile gloves

PROCEDURE FOR VACCINATING NEW EMPLOYEES

1. Define in policy at what point during the orientation process the HBV vaccine will be offered to those employees who have exposure risk

2. Provide the HBV vaccination information sheet to the employee in the orientation packet, noting the following points:

    a. The vaccination requires three separate injections over a specific period of time (the second injection follows one month after the first; the third injection follows six months after the first)

    b. A physician or nurse injects the vaccine into the muscle of the upper arm

    c. HBV vaccine is not effective against any other forms of hepatitis or any other virus that attacks the liver

    d. Following the third injection, the employee will have a follow-up blood test to evaluate the presence of antibodies to the HBV surface antigen (if antibodies are found, the vaccination is considered effective; if the level of antibody is low or a negative titer is found, the employee will receive two booster vaccinations followed by a second blood sample to determine the presence of antibody to the HBV surface antigen)

    e. The employee should have a blood sample drawn again five years following the vaccination series to check for the presence of antibodies to the HBV surface antigen (if the result is negative or shows a low titer, a booster vaccination will be provided)

    f. If interrupted at any point during the administration of this series, the employee may still realize partial immunity to HBV

    g. Allergic reactions to the HBV vaccine are not considered adverse or life threatening and can include redness and/or swelling around the injection site, low-grade fever, and/or flu-like symptoms (all of these symptoms usually resolve within a day or two; anaphylaxis can occur in hypersensitive individuals)

3. Explain to the employee the reason for the vaccination and obtain consent; the only allowable exceptions to the OSHA requirement are:

    a. The employee already had a three-shot series

    b. The employee's antibody titer is up

    c. The vaccine is contraindicated for medical reasons such as pregnancy, immunocompromised status, allergy to yeast, etc.

4. Offer the vaccine:

    a. Free of charge

    b. When it is convenient for the employee to receive the vaccine

    c. Once the employee has received training, but no less than 10 days prior to initial patient contact

5. If the employee refuses to accept vaccination, require him or her to indicate that choice on the appropriate portion of the consent/declination form

    a. The employee should receive a gamma globulin injection in the event of exposure to HBV while performing duties

    b. The employee will require follow-up testing and potential treatment should HBV develop

6. If the employee accepts the vaccination, administer it following established procedure:

    a. Ensure that personnel who administer the vaccine are familiar with general Advisory Committee on Immunization Practices recommendations, well-informed about the vaccine and current on professional recommendations regarding vaccination of healthcare personnel

    b. Define in policy a mechanism to schedule the remaining vaccinations in the series, along with any boosters, if applicable

    c. Develop a mechanism to screen for immunity to HBV within one to two months after the final vaccine dose to persons who perform tasks involving blood, body fluids, and sharps

    d. Develop a procedure to revaccinate persons not found to have an antibody response after the series of vaccines, and obtain follow-up blood tests to determine antibody titers

7. Document whether or not the employee was vaccinated and file in the personnel record

8. Evaluate a process for reoffering HBV vaccine to employees who declined at the time of employment (OSHA guidelines do not define a specific protocol for HBV vaccine, only that one is offered to employees who have direct patient contact—this guideline is based upon the vaccine's manufacturer's guidelines; review the literature to develop a protocol)

Form 4.2: Acknowledgment of hepatitis B information

Employee name: _____ Social Security number: _____

Position: _____ Date of hire: _____

Read the following statements and check the appropriate answer. Provide additional information as requested.	Yes	No
1. I received, read, and understand the information sheet that was provided in my orientation packet regarding hepatitis B vaccinations.		
2. I understand that I am asked to receive the vaccination series because I am at risk for exposure to hepatitis B due to my job responsibilities, and that the vaccine has been developed to help prevent me from getting hepatitis B.		
3. I have been given an opportunity to ask questions regarding the hepatitis B vaccination series and my questions have all been answered.		
4. I understand both the benefits and the potential risks of receiving the hepatitis B vaccination series.		
5. I realize that no guarantee can be made that I will not contract hepatitis B if I receive the vaccination series.		
6. I understand that the vaccination must be given at three different times and that my blood will need to be drawn to test for antibodies. I also understand that if the blood tests reveal the absence of adequate antibody to the hepatitis B surface antigen, I will require one or two booster vaccinations. I will also need a blood test following the booster vaccinations. (Note: Facility policy and manufacturer's instructions dictate whether the facility will test for antibodies.)		
7. I understand that it is my responsibility to keep the appointments set for the vaccinations, boosters, and blood tests. If I cannot keep the appointments, I will notify the agency immediately and reschedule.		
8. I understand that the hepatitis B vaccination series may only protect me for five years, and at that time I will need a blood test to determine the need for a booster vaccination.		
9. To the best of my knowledge, I am not allergic to yeast.		
10. I understand that receiving the vaccinations while pregnant can potentially bring harm to me or my fetus, and I confirm that I am not pregnant or nursing at this time. I further understand that if I should become pregnant at any point in the vaccination series, I must inform the agency immediately so that the vaccinations can cease until such time as I deliver or stop nursing, to be decided by my obstetrician and the manufacturer's recommendations.		
11. I understand that the vaccine can cause complications with some medications and conditions such as treatment for a serious, active infection or compromised cardiac or pulmonary status. I should ask my healthcare provider about any concerns on receiving this vaccination, especially if I have pre-exiting illnesses.		

12. I will immediately inform the physician or nurse administering the vaccination of any change in my health status (including allergies) or any new medications I am taking, whether prescription or over the counter.		
13. I will immediately contact the facility and my personal physician if I experience any side effects from the hepatitis B vaccination.		

Check one box only:

☒ __ I voluntarily consent to receive the hepatitis B vaccination series as it was explained to me above. I release the agency and staff from any liability regarding my decision to receive the hepatitis vaccinations.

☒ __ I refuse the hepatitis B vaccinations offered to me because I already have received my hepatitis B vaccinations.

Date of vaccinations: _____

☒ __ I refuse to receive the hepatitis B vaccination series because _____. I understand that I am at risk for exposure to hepatitis B due to my job responsibilities. I fully accept all consequences of my decision, and I release the facility and staff from any liability regarding my decision NOT to take part in the offered hepatitis B vaccination series.

☒ __ I refuse to receive the rest of my hepatitis B vaccinations because _____. I understand that I am at risk for exposure to hepatitis B due to my job responsibilities. I fully accept all consequences of my decision, and I release the facility and staff from any liability regarding my decision NOT to take part in the offered hepatitis B vaccination series.

☒ __ I understand that I am at risk for exposure to hepatitis B due to my job responsibilities. I fully accept all consequences of my decision, and I release the facility and staff from any liability regarding my decision NOT to take part in the offered hepatitis B vaccination series.

_____

I fully accept all consequences of my decision and I release the facility and staff from any liability regarding my decision to DECLINE the offered hepatitis B vaccination series.

Employee signature: _____ Date: _____

Supervisor signature: _____ Date: _____

Form 4.3: Hepatitis B vaccination record

Employee name: Social Security number:

HBV consent form signed: __ Yes   __ No   Date of hire:

Known allergies:

	Pregnancy status verified verbally/orally	Date vaccinated	Vaccine lot number	Vaccine expiration date	Site of vaccination	Signature
Vaccination #1						
Vaccination #2						
Vaccination #3						
Booster						
Booster						
5-year booster						

Antibody tests

Date:_____ Results: _____

Date:_____ Results: _____

5-year Date: _____ Results: _____

Comments:

SAMPLE PROCEDURE

Tuberculosis Exposure Incident

PURPOSES

- Identify and treat the exposed individual as soon as possible
- Identify the extent to which TB has been transmitted
- Prevent further exposure to healthy individuals
- Demonstrate compliance with OSHA standards for TB controls

SUPPLIES

- TB skin testing materials (PPD solution, alcohol swabs, syringe with needle)
- TB skin testing record (including name, date, method, lot number, date of reading, and size in mm of post-test induration)
- OSHA 300 series form
- Agency-specific reporting form
- Medical follow-up testing and treatment guidelines

PROCEDURE

1. Instruct staff whom to notify immediately if they feel they have been exposed to TB
2. Define and communicate testing and treatment protocol to determine if a staff member has contracted TB and what treatment will follow
3. Establish guidelines on removal from direct patient care until infected individual is no longer considered infectious (this determination is often made following three consecutive, negative acid-fast bacilli smears)
4. Identify an individual to report the exposure incident to the local health department, as well as on the OSHA 300 series form
5. Establish a procedure for notifying and testing any individuals connected with the exposure incident who may also need exposure evaluation
6. Investigate the circumstances surrounding the incident to evaluate whether additional prevention strategies need to be implemented

SAMPLE PROCEDURE

Tuberculosis Exposure Control and Respiratory Protection Plan

PURPOSES

- Take proactive steps toward minimizing exposure to and spread of TB among staff, patients, and family members
- Communicate procedures for staff to follow when they are potentially exposed to TB
- Demonstrate compliance with OSHA requirements
- Provide a protocol for exposure follow-up activities

SUPPLIES

- Binder containing agency respiratory protection plan
- Training program materials
- Skin testing equipment (test solution, syringes, alcohol swabs)
- Personal respirators
- Forms

PROCEDURE

1. Create a protocol for identifying and reporting residents suspicious for signs and symptoms of TB
2. Any new residents admitted should have a chest x-ray completed to make sure they are clear of tuberculosis, regardless of negative PPD results; also, those who have consistently tested positive on the PPD but are not harboring the tuberculosis bacterium should always have a chest x-ray instead of a PPD
3. Create a list of job classifications where there is a potential risk for occupational exposure to TB
4. List the tasks and procedures within each job classification that involve exposure risk
5. Before assigning any staff to patients diagnosed with TB, teach staff how to identify TB, how to prevent the spread of TB, what procedure to follow if exposed, and include:
   a. Epidemiology
   b. Signs and symptoms
   c. Transmission
   d. Risk factors
   e. Work practice controls
   f. Personal respirators
   g. Surveillance
   h. Skin testing
   i. Exposure follow-up protocol
   j. Documentation requirements (OSHA 300 series form)
6. Identify an individual responsible for deciding which staff will wear personal respirators, the type of National Institute for Occupational Safety and Health–approved personal respirators the agency will use, and for teaching staff:
   a. How to fit-test the personal respirator
   b. When to wear the personal respirator

    c. How to inspect the personal respirator

    d. How to maintain the personal respirator

    e. Whom to contact for respirator replacement or repair

7. Create and maintain a log documenting personal respirator training

8. Create and maintain a surveillance protocol for employees, including skin testing for employees and identification of patients or family members suspected of or diagnosed with TB

    a. Perform TB skin tests on employees both pre-employment and according to risk factors thereafter (the most common schedule requires annual skin testing, but tests can occur as often as every three months depending on how many confirmed cases of TB the agency sees annually)

    b. Perform skin testing on residents any time suspicious symptoms are present, but only after consulting with the physician and obtaining an order

9. Establish an exposure protocol for staff exposure to TB and include:

    a. Follow-up testing for staff who test positive during a routine skin test

    b. Whom to contact if exposure is suspected during patient care

10. Establish a procedure for follow-up testing and post-exposure treatment for staff exposed while providing care

    a. Perform a TB skin test on employees as soon as possible after exposure is recognized (except for those known to have a positive test)

    b. Repeat the skin test 12 weeks after exposure (if the test comes back positive, evaluate for active TB; if there is no active disease, consider preventive therapy)

    c. Do not retest employees with reactive tests; conduct follow-up to ensure there are no symptoms

11. Establish procedures for evaluating the circumstances surrounding each exposure incident for purposes of quality (performance) improvement

12. Store the plan where staff can easily access and review it

13. Evaluate and update the plan annually and any time a policy or procedure changes that directly or indirectly affects the original plan

SAMPLE PROCEDURE

OSHA Record Requirements

PURPOSES

- Record the events of any incident when an employee (whether contracted or working directly for the agency) is injured or exposed to an infectious disease such that the employee requires time off from work or has his or her work restricted in any way

- Report any exposure on the OSHA 300 series log:

  —If medical treatment beyond first aid is required

  —That results in seroconversion (to be kept confidential)

  —That is work-related and involves loss of consciousness, transfer, and/or restricted duties

- Make sure every worker injury other than first aid is entered into the log (form 300), and for each worker an injury illness incident report (form 301) should be filled out completely and thoroughly

SUPPLIES

- Recordkeeping system
- Training forms
- Program materials

PROCEDURE

1. Document and file the following information on all staff with occupational exposure to bloodborne pathogens:

   a. The full name and Social Security number of the employee

   b. Copies of the employee's HBV vaccination history from the time of hire to present, including when each vaccination was administered, as well as any other medical records that relate to the employee's ability to receive the vaccination

   c. Copies of the results of all physical examinations, diagnostic testing, or follow-up procedures related to the exposure incident, including HBV and HIV post-exposure test results

   d. The facility/organization's copy of the written report dictated by the healthcare professional responsible for administering HBV vaccinations

   e. Any written reports for evaluation following the exposure incident

   f. A copy of the information sent to the evaluating healthcare professional

2. Maintain confidentiality of all medical information regarding any staff member

3. Disclose information only upon receipt of the employee's written consent, OSHA request, or federal or state laws

4. Maintain training records three full years from the date of each training session, including:

   a. The dates of the training sessions attended

   b. The names and credentials of the trainers

   c. The names and job titles of each staff member attending the training sessions

5. If medical treatment is required, retain medical records, all health-related records, and exposure records for 30 years past the termination of employment

SAMPLE PROCEDURE

Hazard Communication

PURPOSES

- Communicate potential risks to employees
- Develop and disseminate the protocol to communicate that risk to employees who need to know

PROCEDURE

1. Identify and publish a list of conditions and situations that pose harmful risk to staff

2. Complete a material safety data sheet (MSDS or sometimes referred to as the right-to-know) for each hazardous substance used within the agency; make sure all staff are in-serviced on what MSDS is and where it is located for their own information and protection

3. Establish a procedure to inform employees of the risks as they arise in individual resident care situations (this should always be done on each shift among the healthcare workers at the time of shift report.)

4. Assess and educate staff in actions to minimize the risk

Chapter 5

From Theory to Praxis: Staff Education and Competency

Introduction

Care delivered according to infection control guidelines is the most effective tool available for breaking the chain of infection. When implemented properly, infection control practices help stop the spread of infections and promote safe and effective care to residents in long-term care.

Staff education must meet the needs of both the healthcare facility and its staff. A comprehensive educational program begins with policies and procedures. Review the sample procedures in Chapter 4 and modify them to fit your healthcare facility's needs. Then develop a staff education program.

Provide the necessary education and training at the time of hire, especially during new employee orientation, as well as on a regular basis throughout employment. Cover essential components such as universal precautions, infection control techniques, exposure incidents, and regulatory requirements. Focus on the correct ways to perform procedures according to your facility's policies. Maintain careful records so that new employees, contract staff, and even employees with years of experience receive proper training on both existing policies and new procedures. Document the reason for and nature of the content, as well as the attendance at the sessions. Finally, pay attention to supervision. Observe return demonstrations in the classroom and care delivery techniques. Document supervision to show that employees are competent and their performance has been observed and deemed correct by a competent supervisor or instructor.

This chapter is being referred to as "theory to praxis." In the preceding chapters, numerous important concepts were elucidated that need to be understood to carry out a successful infection control program. Those reading this book should have developed an important understanding of the critical concepts presented up to this point. That is the theory component. However, in this chapter, we are now providing a discussion about carrying out this process, especially as it relates to educating and providing a level of competency to your staff. This is the praxis portion. After completing this chapter, readers should have a sound theoretical understanding of infection control for long-term care, as well as a reasonable understanding of how one can inculcate a sound infection control education program for long-term care staff.

In this chapter, you will find many resources to assist you, including:

- Hints for educational sessions that can help you prepare a successful staff education program

- A staff educational program form for documenting education and training

- An outline of a staff educational program that includes key points and guidance for incorporating policies and procedures, Centers for Disease Control and Prevention (CDC) guidelines, Occupational Safety and Health Administration (OSHA) proposed rules, discussion, and practice sessions, and you can expand the outline as necessary and customize to your facility's specific needs by incorporating pertinent policies and procedures and other essential topics that fit with the facility/organization's care delivery practices

- Sample test questions that reflect the content in the educational outline, which you can use in your testing and development

- A chart highlighting the use of personal protective equipment (PPE) that guides staff in planning and delivering care

Staff Competencies Related to Infection Control

A successful in-service program begins with policies and procedures. Once those are firmly in place, plan the content of your in-service education on defining the infection process and ways to contain and control the spread.

New employees who have some experience from other facilities or organizations—or your own experienced employees—may question the need for these sessions or consider them a waste of time. But while infection control is one of those topics everyone thinks they already know, survey citations prove that knowledge is not always put into practice during care delivery. Get staff involved in planning and presenting various portions of the educational sessions; it will stimulate engagement and help break down resistance.

Here are some hints for a successful infection control education program:

- Identify topics to present during orientation and on a regular basis

- Develop a plan for the year

- Schedule in-services at different times to encourage participation and meet the needs of employees

- If you work for a larger company that has several locations, schedule sessions at each of the sites

- Choose instructors who are familiar with the topics and experienced in healthcare delivery; they must teach the classes using language that suits their audience

- Prepare for the sessions; anyone slated to teach the classes must know and understand infection control principles and practices

- Put together an outline and handouts to address the important points in an orderly fashion

- Incorporate visual aids into the sessions

- Focus on facility/organization policies and procedures, as well as specific case studies and examples

- Demonstrate techniques

- Incorporate practice sessions and return demonstrations

- Allow enough time for questions and answers, and if you cannot answer a question, research it and post or distribute the answer

- Teach staff how to fill out forms, such as exposure incident reports

- Create visual reminders with infection control posters, e.g., "Infection Prevention Rocks," "Influenza—An Equal Opportunity Infection," "Sharps/Needles—Handle with Care," "Be Infection Wise—Save Lives"

- Emphasize the need for staff to document observations and actions taken
- Remind staff that infection control practices tend to break down when people become "too comfortable" with a patient or a procedure; stress that being too busy is no excuse for sloppy technique
- Schedule regular follow-up sessions with those employees who request or need additional guidance
- Educational sessions should incorporate opportunities for staff to apply the knowledge they learn; there are several ways to accomplish this
- Discussion sessions bring to light many issues that instructors may not think of when planning the educational programs, so when presenting topics for discussion, use scenarios that play off actual work situations, such as, "What would you do if this happened?"
- When developing test questions, remember that testing evaluates recall of pertinent information (Use the sample questions provided to develop a comprehensive test or quiz)
- Demonstrations and return demonstrations provide the opportunity for staff to gain proficiency right in the classroom, and these practice sessions allow instructors to assess performance and develop follow-up sessions if needed; use the chart provided in this section to discuss PPE during care delivery

Document educational sessions

Document all in-service training in each staff member's personnel file so you have a reliable reference for each employee's status. Develop a one-page format or lesson plan that facilitates quick and complete recording of essential points about the in-service. Include:

- The title of the presentation
- The program objectives
- The name and credentials of the instructor
- The names of any other individuals involved in the presentation
- The content outline, including subject areas, time frames, and methods of instruction
- Resources used
- Summary of discussion, questions, and demonstrations
- Dates and times of classes

The information should adequately describe the subject matter presented and it should demonstrate its relevance for patient care and infection control. Attach handouts, pre- and post-tests, attendance records, and sign-in sheets to the lesson plan. Work with the human resources department to incorporate documentation of participation into individual staff personnel records.

Enlist the expertise of pharmacists, attorneys, or other professionals as resources in planning and presenting in-service programs. Identify ancillary speakers' roles and titles in documentation.

In what follows, you will find a sample form and outline for documenting a staff educational session.

Outline for Educational Session

Outline: The chain of infection	Discussion/notes

To understand why infection control procedures work to stop the spread of infectious diseases, it's important to understand pathogens and how they are spread. In order for diseases to infect a host and survive, they require specific activities to occur and environments in which to live. These events and environments act like the links in a chain. They all need to be present and happen in a specific order for an infection to occur. Breaking that chain at any point prevents the infection.
 	
I. Microorganisms (microbes)
A.   Normal flora:
     1. Thrive in certain areas of the body and serve useful purposes
     2. Can be dangerous if they travel to different parts of the body
B.   Pathogens are microorganisms that cause infectious diseases by entering the body and multiplying
 	
II. Signs and symptoms of infection
A.   Depend upon the type of pathogen, where it is located, and how severe the infection has become
B.   Include:
     1. Fever, chills, or sweating
     2. Headache or stiff neck
     3. Nausea, vomiting, and/or diarrhea
     4. Painful urination
     5. Cloudy, strong-smelling urine
     6. Localized pain or tenderness
     7. Fatigue
     8. Loss of appetite
     9. Rash
   10. Sores on mucous membranes or sore throat
   11. Cough
   12. Localized redness, swelling, or hot sensation to skin
   13. Discharge, drainage (green or yellow, from wound beds)
   14. Crackles, diminished breath sounds, or labored breathing
   15. Rapid pulse
   16. Confusion	

Outline: The chain of infection	**Discussion/notes**

III. The chain of infection
 	
A. The causative agent is the group of pathogenic microorganisms that are carried by the human body and responsible for causing an infectious disease
 	
   1. Protozoa are parasites that live off nutrients in cells and can cause malaria and amebic dysentery
 	
   2. Rickettsia are transmitted by insects and can cause Rocky Mountain spotted fever and typhus
 	
   3. Fungi include molds and yeasts, which can cause thrush, athlete's foot, and allergic or toxic reactions
 	
   4. Bacteria cause a multitude of diseases such as methicillin-resistant Staphylococcus aureus (MRSA), diphtheria, gonorrhea, typhoid fever, tuberculosis, cholera, vancomycin-resistant Enterococcus (VRE), and wound infections
 	
   5. Viruses cause a multitude of diseases such as hepatitis A, B, C, and D; polio; influenza; AIDS; measles; mumps; and the common cold
 	
B. The reservoir is the environment in which pathogens can survive
 	
   1. Human reservoirs include:
      a. A carrier, a person who harbors and can transmit an infectious organism but shows no signs of the disease
      b. An infected person who shows signs of the disease
 	
   2. Animals can also serve as reservoirs
 	
   3. Non-animal reservoirs include street dust, soil, and lint
 	
C. The portal of exit is the pathogens' exit route from the reservoir to infect other hosts
 	
   1. Portal of exit from humans include:
      a. Intestinal tract
      b. Respiratory tract
      c. Genitourinary tract
      d. Lesions or breaks in the skin
      e. Blood or blood products
      f. Semen
      g. Cerebrospinal fluid
      h. Synovial fluid
      i. Pericardial fluid
      j. Amniotic fluid
      k. Other body fluids if they are visibly contaminated with blood, including urine, stool, emesis, saliva, sputum, and wound drainage
 	
   2. Pathogens escape from animals through bites or stings	

Outline: The chain of infection	Discussion/notes

D. The mode of transmission is the method by which pathogens travel from one reservoir to another to spread infection and include:
  1. Direct contact with the infected person
  2. Direct contact with infectious material—for example, nose and throat secretions, blood (bloodborne pathogens), urine, feces, saliva, semen, and vaginal fluids—by activities such as sneezing, coughing, sharing needles, and engaging in unprotected sexual activity; infectious material can also be transmitted in vivo (from within living organism) from mother to fetus
  3. Indirect contact with objects contaminated with secretions, such as dressings, food, needles, or other sharps
  4. Vectors, such as animals, insects, fleas, and ticks
 	
E. The portal of entry is the point where pathogens enter a new reservoir to spread infection—often the same means by which they are able to exit a previous reservoir
 	
F. The susceptible host is a place where pathogens can survive and flourish
  1. Just because a pathogen enters a body does not necessarily always mean the individual will become infected with the particular disease
  2. The body that the pathogen enters may or may not resist the disease; factors that affect resistance include age, immunity, fatigue, general health, medications, nutrition, and drug and alcohol abuse
  3. Individuals at risk for acquiring an infectious disease by a pathogen include:
    a. Those with impaired resistance due to a decreased immune response from conditions such as chronic and/or acute illness, injury, recent surgery, burns, or radiation and/or chemotherapy
    b. Those with high levels of stress
    c. Infants and children
    d. Pregnant women
    e. The elderly
 	
IV. Breaking the chain of infection
A. Breaking the chain of infection in any one place ensures that the infection will either not thrive or not spread
B. Often, the simplest and most effective place to attack the chain of infection is at the potential mode of transmission
  1. Proper infection control procedures will prevent pathogens from spreading
  2. Use proper infection control practices in any situation where the spread of pathogens is possible	

Outline: The chain of infection	Discussion/notes

V. Good personal habits can limit the spread of infection
 	
A. Urge staff to avoid direct patient care if they have signs or symptoms of infection
 	
   1. Since many of the residents' staff care for are susceptible to infection because of one or more risk factors, the infection could be more easily spread
 	
   2. Likewise, an infected staff member is more susceptible to acquiring an infection due to his or her immunocompromised state
 	
B. Stress the importance of keeping clean and practicing good hygiene
 	
   1. Bathe regularly and brush and floss teeth
 	
   2. Keep hair clean and brushed or combed
 	
   3. Groom hair and beard
 	
   4. Wear clean clothing
 	
   5. Trim and clean fingernails
 	
   6. Wear little or no jewelry
 	
C. Protect clothing during care delivery
 	
   1. Hold equipment and linens away from uniforms or clothing
 	
   2. Avoid wearing uniform or work attire at home or out in public
 	
   3. Avoid taking personal belongings into the patient's area
 	
   4. Place care items, on a protectant barrier out of the direct area of care
 	
VI. Employees can take actions to prevent the spread of infection
 	
A. Learn about medical conditions, such as immunosuppression, or medical treatments that render individuals more susceptible to or more likely to transmit infections
 	
   1. It must be emphasized that most residents within long-term care have varying degrees of immuosuppression due to age and poor health
 	
B. Report certain illnesses or conditions, whether they are work-related or not, including:
 	
   1. Generalized rash or skin lesions that are vesicular, weeping, or pustular
 	
   2. Jaundice
 	
   3. Illnesses that do not resolve, such as a cough that lasts two weeks, and hospitalizations resulting from febrile episodes or contagious diseases
 	
C. Follow recommendations on reducing the transmission of infection
 	
D. Cooperate with infection control personnel who are investigating infection outbreaks	

Outline: The chain of infection	Discussion/notes
E. Understand and follow work restrictions relative to certain infectious diseases and conditions F. Evaluate the need for vaccinations; for example, consider requiring influenza vaccine annually to prevent the spread of infection from the flu virus to patients and other staff members	See CDC 2016 Recommended Immunizations for Adults: By Age in reference section

Standard precautions	Discussion/notes
Standard precautions, a key component of hospital isolation precautions, provide guidance for developing an infection control program.	

I. Standard precautions:
A. Are a key component of the CDC's "Guidelines for Isolation Precautions in Hospitals"
B. Recognize the importance of all body fluids, secretions, and excretions in the transmission of nosocomial pathogens
C. Combine the features of:
  1. Universal precautions, which reduce the risk of transmitting bloodborne pathogens
  2. Body-substance isolation, which reduces the risk of transmitting pathogens from moist body surfaces
D. Apply to:
  1. Blood
  2. Body fluids, secretions, and excretions (except perspiration), regardless of whether they contain visible blood
  3. Non-intact skin
  4. Mucous membranes	

II. Key components of an infection control program based on standard precautions include: A. Establishing an exposure control plan with annual updates B. Use of PPE C. Protective housekeeping D. Offering hepatitis B vaccination to employees upon hire E. Offering influenza vaccine to employees annually F. Exposure reporting—keep an up-to-date log of incidents that occur G. Maintenance of employee medical and training records H. Communicating to staff any known hazards	Sample procedures: Personal Protective Equipment, Exposure Incident, HBV Vaccine

Universal precautions	Discussion/notes
The infection control concept that provides the greatest protection from the spread of infection is the practice of universal precautions. These precautions describe protective work practices that should be followed by anyone who comes in contact with a patient.	

I. Key concepts of universal precautions include:
 	
A. Three elements to reflect in facility/organization policy, procedures, and practices:
  1. Consider all patients as infectious and capable of spreading infection
  2. Consider all blood, body fluids, and tissue as contaminated
  3. Consider all used needles and other sharps as contaminated
B. Follow universal precautions when handling any waste—regardless of whether the substance is known to be infected
  1. Infectious waste includes:
    a. Soiled dressings
    b. Used disposable equipment
    c. Reusable equipment that has not yet been cleaned or decontaminated
  2. Infectious waste can be:
    a. Solid (feces)
    b. Liquid (blood, sputum, tears, urine, sperm, vaginal drainage, saliva, wound drainage, irrigated body fluids)
 	
II. The purposes of universal precautions include:
 	
A. Protecting resident, their families and visitors, and healthcare workers from the spread of infection
B. Complying with federal, state, and local laws and regulations, accreditation standards, and OSHA/CDC guidelines
C. Recognizing the risk posed by:
  1. Bloodborne pathogens, such as hepatitis B, hepatitis C, and HIV
  2. TB
  3. Other infectious conditions, such as herpes simplex and Streptococcus
D. Implementing appropriate protective actions
 	
III. Supplies or PPEs to provide protection include:
 	
A. Gloves
B. Masks
C. Goggles
D. Face shields
E. Gowns and aprons (waterproof)
F. Disposable footwear covers
G. Bleach
	Sample Procedure: Hand Washing

Universal precautions	Discussion/notes

H.   Leak-proof containers/red biohazard plastic bags
 	
I.   Biohazard stickers
 	
J.   Sharps containers
 	
K.   CPR devices with one-way respiratory valves
 	
IV. Universal precaution procedures require staff to:
 	
A.   Wash hands
    1. Hand washing with soap and water is the single most effective way to prevent the spread of infection
       a. Since hands are constantly touching contaminated surfaces, they are the principal vehicle for transmitting infection
       b. Follow the healthcare facility's policy and procedures for infection control
       c. Data suggests that a significant percentage of healthcare workers fail to wash hands or follow good technique consistently
    2. Examples of when to wash hands include:
       a. After caring for personal needs, such as using the toilet, blowing nose, covering a sneeze, combing hair, etc.
       b. Before eating, drinking, handling, or serving food
       c. Upon return from public places
       d. Before and after each work shift
       e. Before and after each significant patient contact
       f. Following contact with a contaminated object
       g. After handling waste materials, secretions, drainage, or blood
       h. After handling soiled items, such as linens, clothing, bedpans, urinals, or garbage
       i. Before and after wearing gloves
       j. Before and after touching wounds or performing wound care
       k. Any time contact with infectious material may have occurred
    3. When washing hands, remember:
       a. Liquid soap is preferred, as bar soap kept in a container provides a breeding ground for bacteria
       b. Carry waterless soap or an antiseptic gel hand sanitizer in case there is no running water available
       c. If a towelette or gel is used instead of soap and water, wash hands with soap and water as soon as possible
       d. Carry a supply of paper towels
 	
B.   **Use gloves when there is a danger of contact with blood or body fluids**
    1. Recommended times to wear gloves include when staff are:
       a. Performing mouth care, nasal suctioning, ostomy care, a bowel routine, etc.
       b. Giving enemas
	
	Sample procedure: Gloves

Universal precautions	Discussion/notes

c. Emptying drainage receptacles
d. Performing venipuncture
e. Handling utensils or supplies soiled with body fluids
f. Changing linens soiled with body fluids
g. Cleaning up spills of body fluids
h. Handling specimens
i. Performing wound care or changing dressings (one pair to remove and discard soiled dressing, a second pair to apply new dressing)
2. Gloves are not necessary for casual contact with patients, such as transferring, bathing intact skin, etc.
3. Putting on gloves does not substitute for the need to wash hands
4. Understand latex sensitivity
  a. Many pieces of medical equipment contain latex and may need to be switched to non-latex
  b. Signs and symptoms can range from skin rashes to anaphylactic reaction	

C. Wear protective clothing when there is a chance that blood or body fluids will splash 1. Use disposable waterproof gowns or aprons to protect clothing 2. Use disposable masks to protect mouth and nose area 3. Use goggles to protect eyes 4. Use shoe covers and caps to protect shoes and hair	Sample procedure: Personal Protective Equipment

D. Flush patient wastes (feces, urine, sputum, drainage from suction bags) down the toilet
E. Handle sharps carefully
1. Dispose of used syringes/lancets in the sharps container immediately following any injection or fingerstick testing
  a. The probability of a needlestick greatly increases if staff walk around with the syringe in hand
  b. Avoid recapping needles, bending needles, removing the needles from syringes, or handling them carelessly
2. Carry a spare sharps container in the car in case the patient does not have one
	Sample procedure: Handling Wastes and Disposables

G. Handle specimens carefully as though they were contaminated
1. Follow facility/organization policy and procedure to collect, pack, handle, and transport specimens
  a. Wear gloves when handling the specimen
  b. Keep the laboratory requisition on the outside of the container to prevent contamination from leaks or spills
  c. If transporting a specimen in a facility/organization vehicle, place it on the floor of the vehicle
2. Put specimens in the appropriate leak-proof tubes or containers and then in leak-proof biohazard bags
	Sample procedure: Specimen Collection

Universal precautions	Discussion/notes

3. Never leave needles attached to syringes inside specimen containers
4. The specimens should remain sealed securely until they arrive at the lab
 	
H. Observe sound environmental practices
   1. Follow facility/organization procedure for use, care, cleaning, and storage of equipment
     a. Equipment has great potential to carry and spread infectious material
     b. Whenever possible, use disposable equipment and supplies
   2. Handle soiled linens carefully
     a. Hold linens away from clothing
     b. Do not throw soiled linen on the floor
     c. Avoid fanning or shaking linens
     d. Wash linen soiled with blood or body fluids separately from family laundry
     e. Make sure soiled linen that has blood or body fluids on it is clearly identified for laundry and separated from other dirty linen
   3. Clean up blood and body fluid spills carefully:
     a. Wear gloves
     b. Wipe up spills with paper towels or (preferably) use a blood spill kit; discard properly
     c. Spray area with 1:10 bleach solution or approved disinfectant until glistening wet
     d. Let area dry
 	
I. Follow facility/organization policies and procedures in collaboration with local, and county health department regulations for trash disposal
 	
J. Use disposable resuscitation aids for CPR
   1. Oral barriers or other respiratory protection devices are designed to protect healthcare workers from contracting disease while performing CPR
   2. Both mechanical emergency devices and pocket masks are designed to reduce the risk of exposure from saliva, blood, or other fluids during resuscitation
   3. Follow the facility/organization's procedures for use of mannequins during CPR classes
 	
V. Asepsis and disinfection are important concepts
A. Asepsis refers to the absence of pathogens (disease-causing microorganisms)
   1. The path to asepsis requires two types of actions:
     a. Those that kill or retard the growth of germs
     b. Those that prevent contact with pathogens
	Sample procedure: Handling Linens
	
	Sample procedure: Environmental

Universal precautions	Discussion/notes

2. Aseptic (clean) techniques prevent contact with pathogens by:
   a. Keeping clean and dirty items separated
   b. Working from cleaner areas to dirtier areas
B. Disinfection kills or retards the growth of germs through the use of:
   1. 1:10 bleach solution
   2. 70% isopropyl alcohol
   3. 3% hydrogen peroxide
   4. Some commercial products (Look for wording in the label that describes the product's ability to kill HIV on surface areas treated with solution)
C. Sterilization is a process that kills all microorganisms, both pathogenic and non-pathogenic
D. Know and follow the agency's procedure for disinfecting and sterilizing equipment and supplies
   1. Some instruments can be boiled in water for at least 15 minutes to kill pathogens
   2. Although bleach is an all-purpose disinfectant, it is an oxidizing agent and can corrode met
      a. As an oxidizer it is also harmful to human tissue	

Exposure control plan	Discussion/notes

I. The exposure control plan documents procedures used in controlling exposure to bloodborne or airborne pathogens
A. The purposes of the plan are to:
   1. Communicate procedures for staff to follow when they are exposed to potentially infectious material
   2. Define and communicate steps to take when staff are exposed to pathogens (including but not limited to TB, HIV, and hepatitis) from needlesticks or splashes of blood or body fluids that come in contact with open skin
B. The plan includes essential components:
   1. It promotes communication of hazardous situations to staff ahead of time, when possible (Example: If a patient who is cared for by a staff member has an infection of any kind, communicate that fact, along with the types of precautions the condition requires, e.g., patients who are known to have TB will require staff to wear personal respirators)
   2. It defines and communicates the types of PPE required for all the different kinds of potential infectious opportunities for each patient
   3. It lists those types of jobs where exposure to different pathogens is possible
      a. Staff should follow preventive measures in place (Example: vaccines for hepatitis B and the continuous use of universal precautions)
	Sample procedures: Blood and Body Fluids Exposure Control Plan, Tuberculosis Exposure Control Plan, and Respiratory Protection Plan

Exposure control plan	Discussion/notes

b. The most dangerous potential for exposure comes from those patients who are not yet diagnosed—hence the need to treat all patients as though they are infectious (universal precautions)
4. It addresses TB by describing:
   a. A TB screening program
   b. Management of personnel exposed to TB
   c. Preventive measures
C. **The plan defines ways for staff to handle exposure incidents**
  1. Follow established procedure on steps to take immediately after an exposure to minimize the possibility of becoming infected
  2. Notify the designated individual within the facility/organization following any exposure incident
   a. Know what to do should the exposure occur during on-call hours (Example: Instruct the employee to go to the nearest emergency room for immediate attention)
D. **The plan needs to define the procedures for assessment and treatment of all exposure incidents**
  1. The facility/organization must comply with OSHA requirements regarding follow-up testing, counseling, and post-exposure treatment
  2. Document the incident
   a. Understand the use of the incident report, where it is kept, how to fill it out, and to whom to submit it
   b. The supervisor must notify the facility/organization's infection control manager within 12 hours of the exposure incident
  3. Employees exposed to any infectious disease cannot care for patients until cleared by the infection control manager
  4. If possible, the facility/organization will obtain a consent and test the source's blood, as soon as possible, to identify the pathogen
   a. The facility/organization must reveal the source's test results to the exposed employee, along with disclosure laws and regulations regarding the infected source's right to confidentiality
   b. The facility/organization must document the reason if the source refuses to grant consent for the blood work
 	
  5. The facility/organization will obtain consent and test the exposed employee's blood for HIV and hepatitis B as soon as possible following the exposure incident
   a. The employee may refuse
   b. If the employee refuses to consent to HIV testing but gives a blood sample, retain the sample for 90 days in case the employee gives consent for testing during that time period
  6. The facility/organization must maintain confidentiality
	See CDC-Tuberculosis - NIOSH Workplace Safety and Health
	
	Sample procedures: Blood and Body Fluids Exposure Incident, Tuberculosis Exposure Incident

Exposure control plan	Discussion/notes

II. Exposure incident
 	
A. An exposure incident occurs any time a person comes in contact with blood or a potentially infectious body fluid that can enter the bloodstream through chapped or broken skin, open wounds, mucous membranes, or a needlestick
 	
B. Clean any area exposed to the patient's blood or body fluid immediately, as the exposure can lead to an infection by blood-borne pathogens
 	
   1. If eyes or other mucous membranes are exposed, irrigate with clean water for at least five minutes (make sure your facility/organization has necessary and quickly accessible eye washing stations throughout the facility)
 	
   2. If an exposure occurs in any open cut or sore, wash the area with soap and water and apply first aid
 	
   3. If a needlestick or puncture wound occurs, wash the area with soap and water, Betadine®, or alcohol, and carefully save any sharps or items involved for testing
 	
   4. If any body part is exposed, wash with soap and water
 	
   5. Change clothing immediately if soiled with blood or body fluids
      a. It's always a good idea to keep extra clothing in the car
      b. Wash the contaminated articles in a 1:10 bleach solution
      c. Bag your contaminated clothing in biohazard bag and send to facility laundry for proper sanitary procedure
 	
   6. Notify the clinical supervisor immediately for follow-up instructions
 	
   7. Fill out and submit an incident report
      a. Send the report to the infection control manager within 24 hours of the exposure
      b. The facility/organization will use the information for:
        —Follow-up, surveillance, and evaluation
        —Identifying topics for staff education
 	
   8. Document the entire incident
      a. Include the path of exposure
      b. Unless prohibited by state or local law, identify the name of the infected source
      c. Submit the report to the designated individual
 	
III. Hepatitis B (HBV) and HBV vaccine
 	
A. HBV is a highly infectious virus that attacks the liver
 	
   1. Persons may be at risk for HBV if they:
      a. Have jobs that expose them to human blood
      b. Live in the same house with someone who has a chronic HBV infection
      c. Inject drugs using shared needles
      d. Have unprotected sex with someone infected with HBV	

Exposure control plan	**Discussion/notes**

2. HBV can:
   a. In many cases, cause no immediate symptoms
   b. Be mistaken for the flu due to loss of appetite, nausea, vomiting, joint pain, and mild fever
3. In some of these cases, the disease can go undiagnosed and the individual will become a carrier
4. Most people recover completely from HBV with proper care, enough rest, and a nutritional diet, but some become lifelong carriers
5. There are no drugs that can cure HBV
6. HBV can also cause the following conditions:
   a. Mild illness
   b. Severe illness
   c. Chronic infection
   d. Liver damage (e.g., cirrhosis)
   e. Liver cancer
   f. Liver failure (lethal)
7. HBV is almost 100% preventable with a vaccine
 	
B. **OSHA requires healthcare providers to offer HBV vaccine to employees who are at risk for exposure from infected patients during the performance of their duties**
   1. Providers must offer the vaccinations:
     a. Free of charge
     b. At a reasonable time and place
     c. Within 10 days of initial patient contact
   2. The at-risk population includes healthcare workers who:
     a. Provide direct patient contact
     b. Handle equipment contaminated with blood or body fluid
     c. Collect, transport, or analyze specimens
   3. Employees must know about the vaccinations so they can ask questions before signing the consent form
 	
C. **The agency will schedule a physical and a series of hepatitis vaccinations, as well as antibody blood testing dates (OSHA requires compliance with all items under point B.1, but the facility/organization's policy and vaccine manufacturer's recommendations will dictate whether blood will be drawn for antibody testing following vaccination)**
   1. HBV vaccine is not effective against any other forms of hepatitis or any other virus that attacks the liver
   2. HBV vaccinations require three separate injections over a specific period of time
     a. The second injection is given one month following the first, and the third injection is given six months following the first
     b. A physician or nurse administers the injections into the muscle of the upper arm
	Sample procedure: Hepatitis B Vaccine

Exposure control plan	Discussion/notes

c. The employee should tell the healthcare professional who performs the pre-employment physical or who will administer the HBV vaccination whether he or she recently acquired a new illness or began taking a new medication
 	
3. Following the third vaccination:
    a. A blood sample will be drawn to test for the presence of antibodies to the HBV surface antigen
    b. If antibodies are found, the vaccination is considered effective
    c. If the level of antibody is low or a negative titer is found, the employee will receive two booster vaccinations
    d. After receiving the booster vaccinations, a second blood sample will be drawn to determine the presence of antibody to the HBV surface antigen
 	
4. A repeat blood test should be drawn again five years following the vaccination series to check for the presence of antibodies to the HBV surface antigen (If the result is negative or shows a low titer, a booster vaccination will be provided)
 	
5. If interrupted at any point during the administration of this vaccination series, the employee may still realize partial immunity to HBV
 	
6. The vaccination may present side effects
    a. Allergic reactions to the HBV vaccine are not considered adverse or life threatening
    b. Symptoms include redness and/or swelling around the injection site, low-grade fever, and flu-like symptoms
    c. All of these symptoms usually resolve within a day or two
 	
7. Pregnancy is a contraindication for the vaccine
    a. Since there is insufficient data on the effects of HBV vaccine on a fetus, vaccines are not administered during pregnancy
    b. If the employee becomes pregnant at any point during the series of vaccinations, the series will be discontinued until after delivery/completion of breastfeeding
 	
8. The employee will sign a consent or refusal form
    a. If the employee decides against receiving the required HBV vaccination series and is exposed to the disease while performing his or her duties, he or she will be offered a gamma globulin injection
    b. The employee may also need follow-up testing and treatment, should he or she contract the disease following the exposure incidentSample procedures: Blood and Body Fluids Exposure Control Plan, Tuberculosis Exposure Control Plan, and Respiratory Protection Plan	

Patient with active infections	Discussion/notes
Staff members must practice infection control techniques and universal precautions with all patients, regardless of diagnosis. However, patients with active infections require special care delivery techniques and education.	

I. Patients treated with medications
A. Ensure patients take their medications as directed
    1. Often patients being treated for infections stop taking their medications when they begin feeling better
    2. In order for the medication to prove effective, the full dose is required
B. Encourage adequate fluid intake
C. Report and document any signs of allergic reaction
 	
II. Patients with wound infections
A. Infection control during wound care continues to pose a threat for healthcare workers.
    1. Data suggests that a significant percentage of healthcare workers fail to follow good technique
    2. Teach the importance of consistent, proper infection control practices
B. Staff must understand the signs and symptoms of infection, regardless of their roles in dressing changes. They are:
    1. Redness
    2. Excessive swelling
    3. Tenderness and pain in the area
    4. Red streaks in the skin near the wound
    5. Pus or other discharge from the wound
    6. Foul smell from the wound
    7. Complaints of generalized body chills
    8. Elevated temperature
    9. Increased pulse rate
    10. Enlarged, tender lymph nodes in the area of the wound
C. Pay attention to important practices, including:
    1. Hand washing before and after patient contact
    2. Proper use of gloves
        a. Two pairs may be necessary—one to remove the soiled dressing and a second pair to apply the new dressing
        b. Use non-sterile or sterile gloves as dictated by the procedure
    3. Individualized dressing supplies whenever possible to avoid the potential for cross-contamination
    4. Proper procedure during dressing changes
    5. Properly discarding all soiled disposables (dressings, gloves, gowns, etc.) in a plastic bag, securely closing the bag before disposal
	Sample procedure: infection Control Practices During Wound Care

Patient with active infections	Discussion/notes
III. Patients with AIDS and hepatitis B and C	See Anne Harding and pro and cons of new hepatitis treatments in Reference section
A. Both AIDS and hepatitis B are spread among healthcare workers through:	
1. Accidental sticks and cuts from infected needles or other sharp instruments	
2. Contact with damaged or broken skin	
3. Splashes of body fluids into the eyes, mouth, or nose	
B. Three methods to prevent against these infections are:	
1. Universal precautions	
2. Safe sex	
3. Abstinence from illegal IV drug use and needle sharing	
C. Hepatitis B virus, also referred to as HBV, is a bloodborne pathogen that causes hepatitis B	
1. Hepatitis B is transmitted when blood, blood products, or body fluids contaminated with HBV infect the bloodstream of another person	
2. Hepatitis B is almost 100% preventable with a vaccine	
D. Hepatitis C virus (HCV) is a bloodborne pathogen that causes hepatitis C	
1. HCV infection is the most common chronic bloodborne infection in the United States	
2. Many people infected with HCV are not aware of their infection	
3. There is no vaccine at the present time to protect individuals from HCV infection	
4. However, there has been a recently approved medication for the treatment of Hepatitis C	
E. Acquired immune deficiency syndrome (AIDS) is caused by the human immunodeficiency virus (HIV)	
1. Although great strides in relieving symptoms and prolonging life have been made over the past 15 years, there is still no known cure for the disease	
2. The AIDS virus lives in body fluids and is most commonly spread:	
a. Through sexual contact with an HIV-infected person	
b. By sharing needles with an HIV-infected person	
c. By passing the infection from mother to fetus either before or during birth	
3. AIDS is not spread by:	
a. Donating blood—previously it was, but more advanced screening techniques have allowed this to be highly improbable	
b. Casual contact (e.g., sitting next to, caring for, or shaking hands with an infected person)	
c. Touching something an HIV-infected person touched (e.g., doorknobs, toilet seats, drinking fountains)	
d. Animals	
e. Airborne particles	
f. Food	
g. Kissing	

Patient with active infections	Discussion/notes

IV. Patients with TB
 	
A. OSHA and the CDC require all healthcare workers to follow specific guidelines when caring for patients known to be infected or carrying the disease
 	
B. If an employee who has been occupationally exposed to anyone with a known case of active TB subsequently develops a TB infection, the employer must record the case
 	
C. OSHA requires that the agency provide personal respirators for all staff who may come in contact with a patient suspected of having or known to have TB
 	
    1. Respirators (N95 or equivalent) must have the ability to filter particles of one micron at a filter efficiency of greater than 95%, at flow rates to 50 liters per minute
 	
    2. The healthcare facility needs to evaluate whether there are any employees who, for medical reasons, cannot perform their jobs when wearing a respirator
 	
       a. Staff who are evaluated by a medical professional and deemed unable to perform tasks wearing the personal respirator are exempt from those tasks
 	
       b. Staff who are immunocompromised should refrain from caring for patients who are suspected of having TB or who are diagnosed with TB
 	
    3. The facility/organization will fit-test the employee according to the manufacturer's instructions
 	
a. Fit-test at no greater than 10% face-seal leakage
 	
b. The fit test shall not be conducted if there is any hair growth between the skin and the face piece sealing surface (stubble, beard growth, mustache); any type of apparel interfering with a satisfactory fit test shall be altered or removed
 	
    4. Employees must know:
 	
       a. How to fit-test the personal respirator
       b. How it is positioned on the face
       c. How, when, and why to wear the personal respirator
       d. How to set the strap tension
       e. How to inspect the personal respirator to determine an acceptable fit
       f. How to maintain the personal respirator
       g. Whom to contact for replacement or repair
 	
    5. Monitor the use of respirators in the home environment
 	
D. The healthcare facility/organization should create and implement a TB skin testing schedule per state and/or OSHA guidelines
	See CDC—Tuberculosis—NIOSH Workplace Safety and Health
	
	See Occupational Safety and Health—Tuberculosis—Appendix A on website found in reference section

Patient with active infections	Discussion/notes

1. If a skin test is required due to an exposure incident, the healthcare facility/organization will investigate the circumstances surrounding the incident to evaluate whether additional prevention strategies need to be implemented
2. Follow up according to established procedures
 	
V. Patients infected with antibiotic-resistant organisms
A. The two most common antibiotic-resistant organisms are methicillin-resistant Staphylococcus aureus (MRSA) and vancomycin-resistant Enterococcus (VRE)
B. MRSA is a strain of Staphylococcus aureus bacteria that is resistant to most of the penicillins, cephalosporins, and other antibiotics except vancomycin
  1. It can cause active infections, such as wound infections, urinary tract infections, skin infections, or pneumonia
  2. People without active infection:
    a. Can carry MRSA in the nose or on the skin without any symptoms
    b. Are said to be colonized with MRSA
    —Those colonized are not necessarily showing any types of disease, but can still potentially spread the colonized bacteria to others.
  3. Can transmit the infection from direct skin-to-skin contact or contact with shared items or surfaces that have come into contact with someone else's infection (towels, used bandages, etc.)
C. VRE is an *Enterococcus* that is resistant to most antibiotics, including vancomycin
  1. It can cause active infections in wounds, the gastrointestinal tract, or the urinary tract
  2. People without active infection:
    a. Can carry VRE, usually in the stool, without any symptoms
    b. Are said to be colonized with VRE
  3. It is transmitted from person to person, either on the hands or on contaminated surfaces or equipment
  4. The organism is capable of living for a long time on surfaces such as bed rails or tables
D. Healthcare workers are usually not at risk for infection, but without careful precautions, they can become a link for transmission of MRSA and VRE; they must still adhere strongly to universal precaution standards to prevent causal transmission
  1. Hand washing is the single most important component to preventing the spread of MRSA and VRE
  2. All healthcare staff should focus on prevention of the spread of MRSA and/or VRE by:
    a. Preventing cross-contamination	

Patient with active infections	Discussion/notes

b. Wearing PPE such as gowns, aprons, and gloves when having close contact with infected patients if there are wound exudates, or if contact with blood, stool, or other body fluids may be anticipated
    c. Wearing gloves when cleaning and caring for residents with MRSA or VRE
    d. Cleaning reusable equipment appropriately after patient contact
  6. Infected patients should have their own blood pressure cuffs and stethoscopes and thermometers
E. Teach the patient and family precautions related to MRSA and VRE, including:
  1. Good hand washing techniques and indications
  2. Prompt cleaning and disinfection of bathrooms or other surfaces that may become contaminated
  3. Washing linen heavily soiled with drainage or excretions separately; place in biohazard bag to notify the laundry staff of special precautions and special cleaning methods needed
  4. The need for visitors to wash their hands before leaving the facility to help prevent transmitting MRSA or VRE to others
 	
VI. Teaching tips for all patients
A. Follow proper technique for obtaining, handling, labeling, and transporting specimens
B. Teach each resident, if feasible, how to use their own supplies to prevent cross-contamination.
C. Handle and dispose of infectious material and wastes carefully (e.g., double bagging infectious material for proper disposal and using and disposing within proper identified biohazard container)
D. Follow good personal hygiene practices	

Discussion Topics

Risky patient care scenarios	Discussion/notes
Each of the following situations presents exposure risks for staff members, residents, and others present in the healthcare environment. If you plan ahead and think through a situation, you can minimize the potential for exposure. For each of the following scenarios, discuss the infection control and caregiving actions to take and the use of PPE and supplies. Review healthcare facility/ organization policy and procedures for guidance. Focus on ways to minimize risk and exposure for both the resident and staff while still providing quality care to meet the resident needs.	
A. You must perform venipuncture to obtain a blood sample on a resident who occasionally becomes belligerent and combative B. During the admission visit for a new resident, you are required to administer a one-time dose of an intravenous diuretic C. The resident has HBV; you must feed and bathe them and perform oral hygiene, catheter care, and a bowel routine D. The resident has dementia and experiences both bowel and bladder incontinence; upon arriving at their room, you discover they are not wearing their incontinence brief and have had an episode of bowel incontinence E. You arrive at the resident's room to find they are unconscious and lying in a pool of blood on the floor F. A resident with a tracheostomy is very congested and requires suctioning G. A confused resident needs assistance with oral medication administration; they frequently spit at caregivers as they are administered medications H. The resident has a peptic ulcer; while you take his apical pulse, he begins to vomit I. During rounds one of your residents is experiencing a severe nosebleed; you grab a tissue to hand them and they reach for it with a bloody hand	

Agency policy and procedure	Discussion/notes
Review healthcare facility/organization policy and procedures and discuss the following issues. Add other important topics.	

A. PPE:
    1. Describe the purpose and use of each piece of PPE
    2. Demonstrate the procedure

B. Laundering soiled linens:
    1. Identify the agency's procedure
    2. Describe how to handle soiled linen as it relates for normal dirty linen versus biohazard protocol.
        a. How is linen separated on the basis of different protocol
        b. What type of different cleaning treatment are used
        c. How do laundry workers respond to biohazard linen
        d. They laundry worker have all the necessary PPE readily available

C. Exposure incidents:
    1. Define an exposure incident
    2. Describe the actions to take in the event of:
        a. A splash of blood or body fluid into the eyes
        b. A needlestick with a diabetic patient's used syringe
        c. Bloody wound drainage coming into contact with the caregiver's chapped skin
    3. Describe the healthcare facility/organization policy for responding to an exposure incident and the appropriate follow-up treatment

D. HBV vaccine:
    1. Identify reasons for obtaining the vaccine
    2. Describe the healthcare facility/organization policy on HBV vaccination

E. Respiratory protection program:
    1. Describe the healthcare facility/organization program

Sample Test

Select the answer that best applies.

1. **What is the most effective method of controlling the spread of infection?**

    a. Disinfecting all surfaces with a 1:10 bleach solution

    b. Sterilizing all supplies, linens, and equipment

    c. Hand washing with soap and water

    d. Wearing a mask during all patient contact

2. **How can infection be transmitted during care delivery?**

    a. Through contact with open wounds

    b. Through the patient's linens

    c. Through direct contact with the patient

    d. All of the above

3. **Which of the following diseases is spread by bloodborne pathogens?**

    a. AIDS

    b. Grave's disease

    c. Common cold

    d. Hepatitis B

    e. All of the above

    f. a and d

4. **Which of the following fluids is mostly likely to contain bloodborne pathogens?**

    a. Bloody emesis

    b. Sputum

    c. Drinking water

    d. Vaginal drainage

    e. All of the above

    f. a, b, and d

5. **Which of the following is not a component of standard precautions?**

    a. HIV testing

    b. HBV vaccination

    c. Use of PPE

    d. Exposure reporting

6. **Which statement reflects the principles of universal precautions?**

    a. You can only get an infection from patients with AIDS, HBV, and staph and strep infections

    b. All used needles can cause infection

    c. Only bodily fluids that contain blood can cause infection

    d. All of the above

7. **Which of these practices is dictated by universal precautions?**

    a. Wear gowns and gloves for all contact with AIDS patients

    b. Use a disposable resuscitation aid for performing CPR

    c. Wear gloves to perform oral hygiene on the patient

    d. Do not carry soiled dressings without proper PPEs

    e. All of the above

    f. b, c, and d

8. **When should you wash your hands?**

    a. Before you apply gloves

    b. After handling a bedpan

    c. After arriving at the resident's room and before providing care

    d. All of the above

9. **Which of the following statements describes the appropriate use of PPE?**

    a. Use a specially designed disposable mask to perform CPR

    b. Wear a gown during all patient contact

    c. Wear goggles when caring for the patient with an infectious cough

    d. All of the above

10. **Which of the following procedures does not require the use of gloves?**

    a. Emptying a urinary drainage bag

    b. Preparing the patient's breakfast

    c. Applying a clean dressing to an incision

    d. Performing a venipuncture

11. **Which of these principles appropriately applies to handling wastes and disposables?**

    a. Flush feces down the toilet

    b. Break the needle off a syringe before disposing of it

    c. Double bag all syringes

    d. All of the above

12. **Which of these principles appropriately applies to changing linens soiled with blood?**

    a. Fan and shake linens to remove dust

    b. Throw dirty linens on the floor to avoid contaminating furniture

    c. Hold linens away from your uniform

    d. Launder soiled linens with the family laundry

13. **A portal of entry is:**

    a. where a microorganism is found

    b. where bacteria become colonized

    c. where microorganisms enter into the body

    d. where the infection starts

14. **Which of the following is a recommended practice for disposing contaminated syringes?**

    a. Recap the syringe to limit the spread of bloodborne pathogens

    b. Discard the syringe in one piece to avoid accidental punctures

    c. Use a sturdy cardboard container for disposal

    d. Discard the syringe immediately after injection in the trash in the resident's room

15. **How should you clean up a spill of blood or body fluids?**

    a. Wear a gown, mask, and goggles, and use a sponge

    b. Douse the spill with soap and hot water

    c. Wear gloves and use the facility's approved disinfectant and paper towels

    d. Use a mixture of glycerin and alcohol

16. **Which of the following practices does not appropriately apply to handling specimens?**

    a. Break the needle off the syringe before transporting the specimen

    b. Place the specimen in a leak-proof bag or container

    c. Wear gloves when handling the specimen

    d. Place the specimen on the floor of the facility vehicle if transporting it

17. **What is asepsis?**

    a. A systemic infection caused by asbestos

    b. A no-touch technique for dressing changes

    c. First-aid spray applied to wounds

    d. Absence of pathogens

18. **Which of these is a guiding principle of asepsis?**

    a. Keep clean and dirty items separate

    b. Use a disinfectant solution to bathe your patients

    c. Wear gloves for all patient contact

    d. Work from cleaner areas to dirtier areas

    e. a and d

    f. b and c

19. **Which of these solutions can be used for disinfection of surfaces?**

    a. 1:10 bleach and water solution

    b. Soap and hot water

    c. Glycerin and alcohol

    d. All of the above

20. **What do AIDS and hepatitis B have in common?**

    a. They are caused by a virus

    b. They are bloodborne diseases

    c. They are transmitted through airborne routes

    d. Patients with these diseases must be quarantined

    e. All of the above

    f. a, b, and c

21. **What is HBV?**

    a. High blood volume

    b. A blood test for infectious diseases

    c. Hepatitis B virus

    d. An antibiotic medication

22. **What is one way that AIDS is spread?**

    a. Sharing food with the AIDS patient

    b. Sexual contact with the person with AIDS

    c. Toilet seats in the home of the AIDS patient

    d. Getting bitten by the dog owned by the person with AIDS

    e. All of the above

    f. a, c, and d

23. **What should you do when caring for a patient with active TB?**

    a. Wear an isolation gown and gloves

    b. Wear a personal respirator

    c. Open the window in the patient's bedroom

    d. Let visitors in without masks

    e. a and b

24. **Which of the following is a recommended practice for patients with infections?**

    a. Drink an adequate amount of fluids

    b. Stop taking the antibiotic when you begin to feel better

    c. Use the family towel or drinking glass

    d. All of the above

25. **Which of the following are typical signs of a wound infection?**

    a. Skin that is mottled and cool

    b. Diarrhea

    c. Redness and hotter skin around the wound area

    d. Elevated body temperature and pulse

    e. All of the above

    f. c and d

26. **Which of these principles applies to changing a dressing?**

    a. Wear one pair of gloves to remove the old dressing and put on the new dressing

    b. Don't look at the wound or you may experience nausea and vomiting

    c. Dispose of soiled dressings in a securely closed plastic bag

    d. All of the above

27. **What is an exposure incident?**

    a. An event that you must report to your supervisor as soon as possible

    b. Contact with blood or potentially infectious body fluids

    c. Wearing inappropriate attire in cold weather

    d. a and b

28. **What is the first action to take if blood splashes into your eye?**

    a. Call the nursing supervisor

    b. Apply an antiseptic ointment

    c. Flush the eye with large amounts of clean water, saline, or sterile irrigant

    d. Complete an incident report

29. **Which of the following is not a component of the long-term care facility's exposure control plan?**

    a. A way to limit contact with all patients

    b. A plan to minimize exposure to airborne or bloodborne pathogens

    c. The uniform policy

    d. A plan for respiratory protection

30. **Which of the following factors applies to use of a personal respirator?**

    a. Remove the respirator after leaving the home

    b. The Centers for Medicare and Medicaid Services requires that all employees wear them

    c. Wear one only if the TB patient coughs frequently

    d. Discard the respirator after use

Answers

1.   c – Hand washing with soap and water

2.   d – All of the above

3.   f – a and d

4.   f – a, b, and d

5.   a – HIV testing

6.   b – All used needles can cause infection

7.   f – b, c, and d

8.   d – All of the above

9.   a – Use a specially designed disposable mask to perform CPR

10.   b – Preparing the patient's breakfast

11.   a – Flush feces down the toilet

12.   c – Hold linens away from your uniform

13.   c – where the microorganism enters the body

14.   b – Discard the syringe in one piece to avoid accidental punctures

15.   c – Wear gloves and use the facility's approved disinfectant and paper towels

16.   a – Break the needle off the syringe before transporting the specimen

17.   d – Absence of pathogens

18.   e – a and d

19.   a – 1:10 bleach and water solution

20.   f – a, b, and c

21.   c – Hepatitis B virus

22.   b – Sexual contact with the person with AIDS

23.   b – Wear a personal respirator

24.   a – Drink an adequate amount of fluids

25.   f – c and d

26.   c – Dispose of soiled dressings in a securely closed plastic bag

27.   d – a and b

28.   c – Flush the eye with large amounts of clean water, saline, or sterile irrigant

29.   c – The uniform policy

30.   a – Remove the respirator after leaving the home

Personal Protective Equipment for Patient Care and Contact

Personal protective equipment (PPE) is an important component of the long-term care facility's infection control program. Staff must know how and when to use PPE. Discuss the employee's role in patient care procedures and the type of PPE indicated. Identify when sterile, non-sterile, or utility gloves are appropriate. Evaluate when the employee should wear a gown or apron—the most likely indications are when blood or body fluids are present. Finally, identify situations with the potential for splattering that would indicate the use of a mask or goggles.

Employee Exposure Determination

Staff in the following job categories may encounter occupational exposures to bloodborne pathogens when performing certain duties. Staff should be aware of the exposure risks and use personal protective equipment.

Administrative staff

This includes administrators, clinical directors, clinical managers, and supervisors. In normal performance of duties, these staff are not likely to have occupational exposure. However, if at any time they are performing nursing tasks, they have potential for exposure.

Registered nurses/licensed practical nurses

All have potential for exposure. Examples of duties that may reasonably present exposure risk include:

- Assisting with elimination
- Bathing a patient with open lesions
- Cardiopulmonary resuscitation
- Catheterization
- Dressing changes
- Intravenous infusions
- Invasive tests or treatments
- Irrigations
- Medication administration (IV, rectal, vaginal, inhalation)
- Obtaining specimens (blood, urine, stool, cultures)
- Oral care
- Ostomy care
- Perianal care
- Suctioning
- Tracheostomy care
- Wound care

The following duties do not typically present exposure risk:

- Assisting a patient with ambulation or exercises
- Auscultating heart and breath sounds
- Performing noninvasive treatments, such as pulse oximetry
- Taking vital signs

Certified nurse assistants (CNAs)/personal care attendants

All have potential for exposure. Examples of duties that may reasonably present exposure risk include:

- Assisting with elimination
- Bathing a patient with open lesions
- Cardiopulmonary resuscitation
- Catheter care
- Douche
- Feeding
- Enema
- Linen change
- Measuring output
- Obtaining specimens (sputum, urine, stool)
- Oral care
- Ostomy care
- Perianal care

The following duties do not typically present exposure risk:

- Assistance with ambulation, transfers, or exercises
- Feeding
- Vital signs

Physical and occupational therapists; speech-language pathologists

Some may have potential for exposure in certain circumstances. Examples of duties that may reasonably present exposure risk include:

- Cardiopulmonary resuscitation
- Dressing changes
- Education regarding activities of daily living (e.g., toileting techniques)
- Invasive tests or treatments
- Wound care

The following duties do not typically present exposure risk:

- Assisting patient with ambulation or exercises
- Performing noninvasive treatments
- Taking vital signs

Medical social workers

Some may have potential for exposure in certain circumstances. Examples of duties that may reasonably present exposure risk include:

- Cardiopulmonary resuscitation

The following duties do not typically present exposure risk:

- Assisting with ambulation
- Performing noninvasive treatments

General office staff

None are considered to have potential for exposure during the normal course of their duties.

PERSONAL PROTECTIVE EQUIPMENT FOR PATIENT CARE AND CONTACT

	Hand washing	Gloves	Gown	Apron	Mask	Goggles
Bowel/bladder						
Assisting patient	X	X				
Emptying urinal and bedpan	X	X				
Enema administration	X	X		X		
Manual stool removal	X	X		X		
Ostomy care	X	X		X		
Indwelling catheter						
Care	X	X				
Drainage bag	X	X				
Insertion	X	X	X or X			
Irrigation	X	X		X		
Emergency care						
CPR	X	X		X plus oral barrier		
Hemorrhage	X	X	X			
Superficial bleeding	X	X		X^1		
Feeding tube						
Administration	X	X				
Insertion/removal	X	X		X^1		
Irrigation	X	X		X^1		
Handling wastes and disposables						
Emptying containers (blood, body fluids)	X	X		X		
Handling sharps	X	X				
Disposing of sharps	X	X				
Environmental practices						
Laundry	X	X				
Linen change	X	X				
Spill cleanup	X	X		X^1		
Trash disposal	X	X				
Medication administration						
Intramuscular	X	X				
Intravenous	X	X^2				
Line care	X	X^2				
Line placement	X	X^2	X	X	X	X
Oral	X	X^3				
Subcutaneous	X	X				
Suppository, bowel	X	X		X^1		
Suppository, vaginal	X	X		X^1		
Topical	X	X				

	Hand washing	Gloves	Gown	Apron	Mask	Goggles
Personal care						
Bathing	X	X[4]				
Feeding	X	X				
Oral hygiene	X	X				
Perineal care	X	X				
Specimens						
Blood	X	X	X[1]	X[1]	X[1]	
Sputum	X	X	X[1]		x1	X[1]
Stool	X	X	X[1]			
Urine	X	X	X[1]			
Temperature, rectal	X	X				
Treatments						
Fingerstick blood glucose	X	X				
Respiratory	X	X[2]	X	X[1]	X[1]	X[1]
Suctioning	X	X		X[1]	X[1]	X[1]
Tracheostomy care	X	X		X[1]	X[1]	X[1]
Urine testing	X	X				
Venipuncture	X	X		X	X	X
Wound care						
Dressing change	X	X	X[1]	X[1]		
Irrigation	X	X	X[1]	X[1]		X

[1] Use and choice of personal protective equipment is determined by the situation. Is there a possibility that blood or body fluids will splash or spatter?

[2] Use of non-sterile or sterile gloves is determined by the procedure.

[3] Wear gloves if placing medication in the patient's mouth.

[4] Change gloves PRN soiling.

Infection Control Competencies

The goal for every healthcare worker is competency in infection control techniques. To achieve that goal, the long-term care facility must provide staff education, as well as opportunities for demonstration and practic; education by itself is not enough. Infection control breaks down when a long-term care facility provides the education and then assumes its staff is following procedure. As the survey citations point out, this is a dangerous assumption to make. There are three essential steps to carry out after the education is completed:

- Assess educator and trainer competency
- Assess employee competency
- Supervise employees

Assess educator and trainer competency

- Make sure that the trainer or educator has attended proper education on infection control.
- Make sure he or she has a proper level of credentials for this area, such as coursework that has been regularly taken in this area, or certifications achieved from meeting certain education requirements.
- Do not think that just because a person is a licensed healthcare worker, he or she knows and is able to provide proper instruction on infection control
- Make sure the individual who is conducting infection control education has proper documentation, that attests to his or her ability to have a sound education of infection control, such as a certificate or diploma.
- Attend the instructor's class and make sure he or she is carrying out classes in an organized and educationally conducive manner.

Assess employee competency

This list should guide your documentation of education, demonstration sessions, and actual in-facility observation.

- Instruct the employee to complete the self-assessment component. This will provide some insight into his or her educational needs.
- Record the date of education training, and demonstration sessions.
- Record the date and pertinent comments related to return demonstrations in the classroom or in-home observation.
- Document any comments.
- Follow up on any significant findings.
- If more than one instructor or supervisor participates in the education and supervision, each should initial the entries and sign the form. Use this form at the time of orientation and periodically throughout employment to reassess performance.

Supervise employees

Measure the ongoing effectiveness of your infection control education by adopting routine supervisory observations of staff providing care to residents within your facility. During these visits, you can monitor infection control as well as other aspects of care delivery.

If periodic supervisory observation is new to your professional staff, employees may become resentful or anxious. Address these feelings by helping staff understand the reasons for the observation.

If staff members become accustomed to being periodically observed by supervisors during care delivery by supervisors, it will put them more at ease when being observed by surveyors. That means they should make fewer "nervous mistakes," such as forgetting to wash their hands. In this era of intense scrutiny, it is essential that the long-term care facility is proactive (preventing problems before they occur) rather than reactive (enforcing policy only after a citation has been issued).

The goal of supervisory observation is to ensure the infection control procedures really serve their intent—keeping the staff, residents, and patients' family members from spreading infection. The observational visits may turn up some problems in practice, which will allow the long-term care facility to modify the procedures accordingly. To ensure appropriate supervision, teach supervising staff what to look for while observing staff during care delivery. Reinforce documentation requirements, and how to determine when additional training and supervision is necessary.

INFECTION CONTROL COMPETENCIES

Employee name: _____ Date of employment: _____

	Self-assessment		Education	Demonstration	In-home observation	Comments
	Need review	Competent				
Nursing bag technique						
Bowel/bladder						
Assisting patient						
Enema administration						
Manual stool removal						
Ostomy care						
Hand washing						
Indwelling catheter						
Catheter care						
Drainage bag						
Insertion						
Irrigation						
Emergency care						
Hemorrhage						
Superficial bleeding						
Feeding tube/ G-tube placement						
Administration of meds/feeding						
Insertion/removal of feeding tube						
Irrigation						
Environmental practices						
Laundry						
Linen change						

	Self-assessment		Education	Demonstration	In-home observation	Comments
	Need review	Competent				
Sharps handling and disposal						
Spill cleanup						
Waste disposal						
Medication administration						
Intramuscular						
Intravenous						
Central line care						
Line placement						
PICC line care						
Subcutaneous						
Suppository, bowel						
Suppository, vaginal						
Topical						
Oral						
Personal care						
Bathing						
Feeding						
Oral hygiene						
Perineal care						
Personal protective equipment						
Sterile gloves						
Non-sterile gloves						
Utility gloves						
Face mask						
Face shield						
Goggles						
Gown						
Apron						
Disposable CPR mask						
Personal TB respirator						
Specimens						
Blood						
Sputum						

	Self-assessment		Education	Demonstration	In-home observation	Comments
	Need review	Competent				
Stool						
Urine						
Temperature						
Treatments						
Fingerstick blood glucose						
Respiratory						
Suctioning						
Urine testing						
Venipuncture						
Wound care						
Dressing change						
Irrigation						
Negative pressure wound vac						

Comments: _____

_____

_____

_____

_____

_____

_____

Employee signature: _____ Date: _____

Supervisor signature: _____ Date: _____

Chapter 6

Patient Education

Introduction

Your infection control program won't be complete without resident and family caregiver involvement. They must know about and practice infection control techniques to protect themselves. One may ask: why do residents and family members have to learn about infection control in a long-term care facility? Is that not what they are there for—to be taken care of? Yes, this is true. However, since many residents (notice the term, residents) will adopt these facilities as their new homes, and since they will be living in close contact with others, the potential to spread infection is great. Furthermore, since many individuals in long-term care environments are older and somewhat immunocompromised, family members should be aware that they can be potential hosts and, as infectious agents, can pass microbial elements that they come into the facility with to others.

One does not expect residents and family members to understand the intricacies of infection control to the same level as professional staff. Yet, making sure you constantly are educating, shaping, and reinforcing their understanding in this area can aid you, the healthcare professional, in your quest for enhanced infection containment and control. Plan, implement, and evaluate an individualized teaching program to meet the patient's needs and abilities. The teaching sessions must suit the level of comprehension of each individual resident and family member.

In this chapter, you'll find resources to help you plan, implement, and document a teaching program, including:

- Adult learning principles
- Tips for teaching older adult patients
- General infection control principles
- A teaching program on infection control

Teaching Your Patients

Adults bring a lifetime of experience to the learning situation, and most of them are capable of self-direction. They often relate the development of new skills to competencies they learned in their occupational and social roles. Build on those experiences. They provide a useful connection between their past and their present situation. Building on their prior experience also shows respect for the resident, builds rapport, and trust. Successful instruction depends on an accurate assessment of the resident's needs, an individualized teaching plan, comprehensive teaching strategies, and evaluation.

Assessment is the first step in resident education. Evaluate your residents' skills and knowledge in important areas. Consider their reading level, ability to learn, and ability to understand English, and use specific resources available to them. Use the findings from your assessment to develop a unique plan for the resident. For instance, a resident who is a retired nurse with experience in infection control is already going to have a sound base on which to build. Conversely, a person with severe cognitive deficit is probably not an individual who will garner much success from education and instruction.

Most adults like to apply new information quickly. They may not get things right the first time, but each mistake provides an opportunity to learn. Give residents the opportunity to take the lead, again reinforcing respect and trust.

Invite family caregivers to be part of your infection control teaching process. At teaching sessions, you can further assess family dynamics. If one of your goals is to promote resident independence, make sure family members understand that their role is to support the resident in this area, and they should not take over tasks that the resident is able to do on his or her own. Conversely, if your goal is to teach family members infection control practices that they should follow for a family member who has a severely immunocompromised status, make sure that they understand it will become their responsibility to provide safeguards to protect themselves against infections and that frequent hand washing is also necessary for them when they interact with their family member even on a casual basis. Moreover, encourage family caregivers to review and frequently reinforce what the resident is learning to assist in providing a well contained infection control environment

Remember that one of the goals of long-term care is to prevent those in nursing care facilities from having any unnecessary or unanticipated declines. Furthermore, residents should attempt to remain as independent as possible. This includes being able to assist and advocate in their care. That being said, there are some individuals who will be able to be more independent in their daily activities than others. They may meet the required OBRA standards to be a resident in a long-term care environment, but they may also want to be involved in caring for themselves as much as possible. These individuals may be amenable to education and teaching in this area. For instance, teaching ostomy care to the resident if he or she chooses to apply what he or she has learned, enhances self-confidence and independence, and, quite frankly, it helps out the staff as well. However, it must be done correctly and follow proper infection control procedures—a resident who just takes off an ostomy bag and puts on a new one, leaving the old one open and airborne, does nothing to minimize the infection control risk and actually increases it. So if a resident wants to assist in his or her own care, make sure infection control procedures are followed correctly.

Teaching any individual is a challenge and teaching individuals who may not be in the best of health, and may even have some memory issues, will need considerable follow-up and reinforcement. Your teaching plan will likely require more than one session. The sessions should contain some overlap so the patient can logically connect the steps covered in each session. Conclude each session with a review of the material you have covered and your goal for the next session. Use a summary session to facilitate the process of integration and to allow for evaluation and feedback. Make sure the resident, after being shown the procedure, is able to demonstrate it to you. Always make sure your instruction is concise, clear, and simple. The slightest ambiguity can cause failure in resident education. Do not hesitate to place reminders in conspicuous areas, such as hand washing posters by the sink to remind residents to always wash their hands thoroughly for at least 20 seconds with soap and warm water.

Tips for teaching the elderly resident

Many of your residents will be over the age of 65. Residents of this age group will need a slightly different approach to meet their learning needs effectively. In fact, Malcolm Knowles (1984) developed the theory of andragogy, as opposed to more pedagogical youth-based learning approaches. According to Knowles, adult individuals learn best when things are practical and relevant to their needs in life. Teaching and educating adult residents should be based on this premise. Consider the following tips for teaching residents:

- Maintain a positive attitude. Treat the older adult as intelligent and capable of learning.

- Take a few minutes to talk and problem solve before starting to teach. Ask the resident about his or her experience in a given area. Find out what has and hasn't worked in the past.

- Identify significant cultural or social factors that may affect the teaching and learning process.

- Include the patient in setting learning goals. Keep the material relevant to the learner's needs.

- Identify and try to accommodate any disability that may affect the learning process. For example, for patients with visual impairment, encourage the use of glasses (if appropriate) and investigate special learning tools, such as large-print material.

- Slow the pace of instruction and gear teaching to the patient's rate of absorption. Stop teaching if the patient appears tired or stressed.

- Break each topic into small parts. Repeat sessions when necessary. Give pertinent, positive feedback.

- Ask the patient to talk through the procedure before trying it. Provide opportunities for practice sessions and repeat demonstrations. Avoid tests or challenges—these are residents, not students. You are attempting to make sure they understand important principles of infection control to help them. You are not attempting to make them into an infection control expert.

- Assess responses carefully to make sure the information was understood correctly. Gear the frequency and duration of your teaching to match your resident's learning ability and need to know.

- As previously stated, add cues or reminders within the environment to help remind them about important infection control practices, such as hand washing posters above the sink.

Document resident education

To support teaching, record the resident's knowledge and skill deficits in the clinical record. Note any limitations that may affect the educational program. This is also very important if some residents are there for short-term rehabilitation and may end up returning to their residence outside of the facility. Your clinical evaluation should always anticipate that they may leave, and important skills and training that the resident may need to know to enhance proper infection control procedures are imperative for their discharge.

Document the teaching plan, noting short-term goals, resources and materials used, and specific interventions. Record actual instruction and describe the patient's response. When teaching is completed, summarize the patient's progress by describing modifications in the patient's behavior (e.g., "Patient demonstrates correct dressing disposal technique"). Explain reasons why the patient may not have learned.

General Infection Control Principles Within the Healthcare Facility for Homebound Residents

Infection control issues in the healthcare facility pose special challenges. As mentioned, many residents (in fact an ever-increasing amount of both middle-age and older adults) are now coming to long-term care facilities for short-term rehabilitation and will need education in many areas, including infection control, to assist them in their care when they are discharged. It's important to educate the patient and family caregivers on ways to reduce infection. Infection control for these individuals can be divided into four parts:

- The environment
- Personal hygiene and nutrition status
- Treatments
- Universal precautions

Environmental infection control

Teach patients and caregivers how to keep their environments (including their homes if they are discharged) clean, leading to a reduced likelihood for infections to happen. Demonstrate how they should be vigilant in addressing the following:

- Wipe items that are used for meals or snacks, such as tray tables or trays attached to wheelchairs, with soap and water after each use.
- Keep kitchen eating and food preparation surfaces clean.
- When preparing food, avoid using wooden cutting boards, especially for meats, because the cracks in the board harbor harmful bacteria, such as Salmonella and E. coli.
- Wipe counters and cutting surfaces immediately after use with a bleach solution or commercial disinfectant. (Long-term care facilities may actually have simulated kitchen and dining areas as part of their PT/OT rehabilitation when they know they will be sending residents back to their former environments. These types of settings are excellent areas to inculcate the importance of infection control procedures).
- Clean bathrooms regularly, especially if these are places where they may be doing such things as ostomy care.
- Wash vinyl or tile floors weekly with a commercial disinfectant.
- Wash plastic trash containers weekly with soap and water, then spray the inside with a commercial disinfectant.
- Clean medical equipment according to the manufacturer's instructions.
- Launder linens soiled with blood or body fluids separately.
- Clean spills of blood or body fluids with a 1:10 bleach solution or a commercial equivalent. Wear utility gloves for these types of chores, and clean the gloves with soap and water when finished.
- Explain how to bag soiled dressings or other potentially infectious material in a disposable leak-proof bag, double bagging it if the material is soiled considerably and is capable of leaking, and then placing in a labeled biohazard bag.

Include family caregivers in the education sessions, if necessary. Some residents, including those who are quite independent, may be going back to live with a family member. In this case it is often important for family members to have some level of infection control education as well. Whether it is the single resident or the resident and their family members, they all must know the proper actions to take and personal protective equipment to wear when providing care. For example, they should wear disposable gloves when handling or coming into contact with blood or body fluids. Even the resident, who may be providing care to themselves, should be aware that they need to use gloves or use other infection control protocols on themselves to prevent introducing infectious agents.

Family members who are involved in assisting in the care of a homebound resident should be trained and educated on such things as where and how to dispose of needles and syringes, such as for those who are diabetic. They should also be instructed on proper disposal of biocontaminants, such as tubing, dressings, blood and blood product stained laundry that may need to be disposed of.

Personal hygiene and good nutritional status for infection control

Teach patients and caregivers that keeping clean and eating right is their best defense against infection. Remind them to:

- Use liquid soap in the bathroom. Teach proper times and methods of hand washing, and the importance of washing hands often, especially prior to, and after, rendering care to themselves.

- Wash clothing, bedding, and towels regularly.

- Bathe, shower, or wash regularly. Cover wounds as prescribed by the physician to avoid trauma to the area or loss of new tissue granulation.

- Never share toothbrushes, handkerchiefs, drinking glasses, eating utensils, or dishes, especially with those who are already immunocompromised or may be on immunocompromising agents, such as high levels of corticosteroids or agents such as cyclosporine.

- Cover mouth and turn away from others when sneezing or coughing.

- Refrigerate perishable foods; discard items that are past their expiration date. This is important to emphasize. Many older adults, especially those on a limited income, will continue to use, heat, and reheat perishable food items well beyond healthy time periods.

- Eat a balanced diet, drink plenty of fluids, and try to get enough exercise and rest.

Receiving adequate treatment

Residents and family members should see a physician regularly to establish a baseline medical history and relationship for future treatment. Instruct patients and their family members to:

- Take medications as prescribed.

- Perform medical treatments as prescribed using aseptic techniques. (Incorporate frequent practice and demonstration sessions.)

- Ask their physicians about immunizations.

- Recognize the signs and symptoms of infection to take prompt action. Among those that go home and will take on the duties of their own care afterward, this is critical. They must be fully informed about checking for infection regularly. During the period of convalescence, they may be gaining some strength, but they are still highly susceptible to infection. A small infection that is dismissed can quickly become a larger generalized septic infection and can quickly lead to rehospitalization, readmission to a long-term care facility, or, even worse, death.

  — The important signs and symptoms they should be instructed to look for daily are: fever, chills, or sweating; headache, stiff neck, nausea, vomiting, and/or diarrhea; painful urination or cloudy, strong-smelling urine; local pain or tenderness; fatigue; loss of appetite; rash; sores on mucous membranes or sore throat; cough; local redness, swelling, or hot sensation on skin; discharge or drainage (green or yellow from wound beds); crackles, diminished breath sounds, or labored breathing; rapid pulse; and confusion.

- Call their physicians immediately if they experience any of the signs and symptoms of a medical problem or infection.

Universal precautions

Teach patients and family caregivers that following universal precautions is the best defense against acquiring infectious diseases. Caution them to:

- Treat all blood and body fluids containing visible blood as though they are contaminated. (Fluids in the womb, semen, and vaginal secretions, as well as fluids surrounding the heart, lungs, brain, stomach, joints, and tendons, are all capable of carrying viruses.)

- Wear gloves or other protective clothing when handling specimens or coming in contact with blood or body fluids. This includes even those individuals who are providing care to himself and may be providing wound care. Advise them to protect the eyes, nose, and mouth if there is a possibility of contaminated fluid splashing into the face. Also advise the resident who provides care for themselves to avoid touching other areas of the body, such as scratching the eyes or nose, after providing care to such things as wounds unless they have thoroughly washed their hands.

- Wash hands often, especially after handling any blood or body fluids, before and after handling food, or using the bathroom. This includes those who are providing care to themselves.

- Cover any broken skin with a bandage or dressing.

- Dispose of sharps carefully, taking care not to touch the needles. Use a regular biohazard container or a hard plastic, sealable container for disposal.

- Clean up any blood or body fluid spills immediately. Wear gloves and use paper towels. Disinfect the area with a properly approved product or 1:10 bleach product. Wash soiled linens immediately. Avoid touching the linens on clothing or other surfaces.

- Practice safe sex.

- Use needles only once.

Chapter 7

Quality Improvement and Infection Control

Introduction

The last component to an effective infection control program is a method to ensure the agency identifies and reduces the risks of infection for residents, caregivers, and visitors who enter the healthcare facility. That is where quality improvement (QI), also known as performance improvement, comes into play. An effective QI program should incorporate measures for surveillance, prevention, and control of infection. State and federal government regulations, accreditation organizations, and standard practice guidelines all demand these measures.

Although the governing bodies and accreditation organizations do not propose any specific approaches to meet infection control requirements, they do expect to see clear evidence that agencies aggressively seek to minimize the spread of infection. Consistent use of infection control techniques, as well as efforts made to educate patients and family caregivers, serve this goal.

In this chapter, you'll find information to help you effectively integrate infection control into a QI program, including:

- A discussion of how the healthcare facility/organization QI program incorporates measures for surveillance, prevention, and control of infections
- Ways to track and trend infections
- An explanation of the complexity of finding cause
- A brief introduction into some statistical techniques to improve your infection control QI

The Role of Infection Control in Quality Improvement

Three key elements of an effective infection control program are: surveillance, prevention, and control of infection. The agency's QI program plays an important role in all of these elements.

Surveillance is defined as "a watch kept over a person, a group, etc." More specifically, surveillance is continuous, systematic collection, analysis, and interpretation of health-related data, not only within your healthcare facility, but outside of it as well. In an infection control program, the healthcare facility/organization can collect data about infections to identify trends, patterns, or problems, and this can go in a number of different directions.

1. Collect data about every infection that occurs within the long-term care environment. (This method of surveillance works best if the healthcare facility/organization is smaller or experiences a low number of infections).

2. Collect data about specific patient populations or procedures (e.g., residents who develop UTIs).

3. Collect data about high-incidence populations or procedures (e.g., seven staff members develop staph infections in one week).

4. Document infections that occur within a particular period of time or particular location in a given healthcare environment.

5. Document efficacy of treatment and any evidence of antibiotic resistance.

The healthcare facility/organization must have a method to identify infections. The following sources provide useful information for tracking and trending (although not necessarily the most empirical or scientifically quantifiable information) for QI studies:

- Infection reports
- Infection report log
- Incident reports
- Workers' compensation claims
- Exposure incident reports
- Clinical records
- Personnel records
- In-service records

Your long-term care facility's QI team may identify other sources of data for its studies. Surveillance serves an important role in quality investigation or quality assessment, the first component of the QI process. Remember that good QI surveillance does not just focus on the internal long-term care environment; it also focuses on the environment outside of your organization. Infectious agents that exist outside of your building's foundation can still play an important role in affecting your internal resident and worker environment. For instance, think about our annual influenza issues. Although they may not have penetrated your resident environment, the first occurrences in the community around your healthcare facility could be a very important "call to arms" for the QI infection control committee to address the potential impact on their resident and worker population.

Excellent surveillance is imperative for helping to direct infection control efforts, especially on a preventative means. Once your surveillance has identified important or impeding issues, the QI committee or team can structure and conduct further investigation into potentially pressing infection control issues. After identifying the area of focus, the committee would determine the methodology (data that are collected, data sources, who is responsible for reviewing and analyzing the data), evaluate the results, and identify actions to improve care. Further on in this chapter, a discussion will be provided on how a long-term care environment can improve the quality of their investigation as it relates to infection control.

After completing the initial QI efforts, the healthcare facility/organization must take action to ensure that improvement is sustained. For the infection control program, that would mean taking action to prevent the occurrence of infections and prevent the spread of infection to and from residents, staff, and visitors. QI and infection control work together to reduce and control infections through enhanced training, technical innovation, and improved procedures.

As a healthcare provider, your healthcare facility/organization is responsible for:

- Ensuring that all staff know and use current best practices to ensure they are not spreading infection while providing care
- Educating families and other caregivers on best practices for the control of infections within your healthcare environment (e.g., do not visit if you are sick)
- Tracking and trending infections
- Implementing measures to improve the quality of care and services provided

The committee can develop the following methods to ensure the agency's infection control program meets its objectives:

- Identify problems related to risks and hazards
- Implement action plans to eliminate or reduce risk
- Monitor and evaluate effectiveness
- Identify and resolve potential risks before someone is injured
- Review potential claims and significant incident reports and trends
- Monitor risk compliance with regulatory agencies
- Analyze risk management concerns and recommend solutions
- Review and revise policy
- Develop and present staff educational programs

Tracking and Trending Infections

The only way to ensure your infection control program is effective is to assess its efficiency on an ongoing basis. Your program might sound pretty good on paper, but is it really preventing the spread of infection to residents? One way to measure the efficacy of your infection control program is to track and trend patient infections. With the help of some basic data gathering and analysis tools, you can begin to quantify effectiveness.

Before you begin examining your data, spell out exactly what it is you want to know. For this exercise, assume you are only concerned with preventing residents from contracting infections while receiving services within your long-term care facility.

First, you will need some mechanism for collecting data on resident infections. One option is a patient infection report. Here's how it works: Your nurse or therapist completes a patient infection report for any patient with an infection, which then becomes a part of the patient's clinical record. The form should allow you to separate infections that were evident on admission from infections that the patient contracts while in the healthcare facility. For purposes of the data described here, you would only count the infections that were contracted while within the care of the long-term care facility—not infections that were evident on admission. Something to take note of: clinical research suggests that any infection that occurs within 48 hours after hospital discharge should be considered nosocomial, that is, a hospital-acquired infection. This can be an ambiguous area, so your form should have a section that reflects possible hospital acquired/nosocomial infection. On a regulatory level, surveyors may view it as an infection acquired within the facility if it first manifested in your long-term care facility. Without any definitive proof of any source of infection, any exact microbial specimen, or any knowledge regarding transfer from point A to point B, the exact causative agent of where and when the infection was acquired will be dubious at best. The next step in the process of self-monitoring is to "trend" infections that occur and then analyze those trends in an attempt to determine their causes.

By completing a resident infection report when the signs and symptoms of infection are present, the long-term care facility can keep track of infections. In order to facilitate analysis of that data, records of infections need to be compiled and organized. One way to do this is to have the infection control nurse(s) or proxy write the relevant information from the individual resident infection reports on the resident infection log. Data on all infections should be kept daily. They should specify the signs and symptoms of the infection, the physician diagnosis of the infection and particular diagnosis provided, where in the facility (room, floor, hallway, etc.) the infections were found, they type of treatment that was provided, efficacy of the treatment, as well as any suspected resistance that may have been documented to any type of antibiotic therapy. The infection control nurse should provide a monthly report on the number and types of infections that were found in the facility for a given month and how it compared to previous months. The use of simple descriptive statistical tools such as bar graphs, histograms, Pareto diagrams, or box plots can aid in examining these trends within the facility. In fact, even using a diagram of the facility and using dots to place the location and types of infections can provide a very nice visual examination of the spread of containment that exists on an infection control level.

After organizing and collecting the data, the infection control committee determines whether a change in the infection control program is warranted. If very few patients are contracting infections, perhaps the program is fine the way it is. But if the committee believes the number of patients contracting infections is too high, then the next step is to analyze more specifically the infections that are being found within the facility. The committee looks at a number of variables, including:

- Which patients are contracting infections
- The types of infections
- The circumstances surrounding the cases of documented infections
- Locations of where infections are being found in the facility
- Levels of care that is needed by residents experiencing various types of infections
- Level of potential immunocompromised status
- Whether the infection is preventable or not given the status of the resident

In analyzing these variables, the committee will try to determine the contributing factors or cause of the infections. An emphasis must be placed on the word try. In reality, most elements of cause are difficult to isolate. The reason for this are: (1) individuals are notoriously poor at causal analysis; most individuals have very little, if any training, in this area; (2) in most long-term care settings, the availability of resources to achieve specimen isolation is problematic and quite limited; (3) in many cases a correlation can be found, but not necessarily a cause; and (4) often the cause is not singular, but multifaceted. Nevertheless, as an analysis is undertaken, it may show that infections are related to poor technique, resident noncompliance with drug therapy or other forms of treatment, or patient conditions in general. If the committee, for example, identifies poor field technique as a possible cause of the infections, education and supervisory observation are actions you can take to address this cause.

If you examined your data, isolated an issue, educated your staff, and engaged in supervisory observation and follow up but no effect was found to limit infections, reevaluate the need for such interventions. Consider what other causes, besides sloppy infection control practices, may be causing the infections. Individuals are novices at casual analysis. You may have found one agent that is instrumental (causative) in the infection process, but not the only agent. Many individuals go into an analysis often quite naively, seeking to find a single cause when, in fact, there are multiple agents contributing to the problem. This is more often the reality! However, our need to reduce and simplify will at times make us fail to see that many things are contributory agents to the issue we are attempting to solve. Also, we must remember that what we think is the cause may actually not be. Therefore, regardless of how well our program works for eliminating or correcting the infection control issue, if we have found or isolated the wrong issue, our solutions, no matter how well-organized, structured, and focused they are, will not work.

Examining Cause

It was mentioned above that one of the major errors individuals make is in the use of causal analysis. As was mentioned, individuals often make mistakes in (1) assuming that there will always be a "findable" cause, (2) thinking there is only a "single" cause, (3) failing to adequately "isolate" the real cause if one is found, and (4) failing to acknowledge that the best one can find may be a "correlation" rather than a cause. Mistakes of causal analysis often occur due to inappropriate training and a lack of understanding about how to undertake such an endeavor. Therefore, more time must be spent addressing the topic of causal analysis. Furthermore, understanding some important concepts of causal analysis is imperative in any form of QA/QI process, including those related to infection control.

We may say that there is an ultimate cause to everything, but often an ultimate cause will never be found. In reality, most causal analysis that we do find is not made up of a single cause, but multiple causes. Say, for instance, a person comes down with the influenza virus. This person is 85 years old, had cancer, was immunocompromised, and had a visitor who was showing symptoms of the flu. What was the cause? Good question. Most healthy individuals who interfaced with the person that harbored the virus never did get sick. So, was it the person's age or their immunocompromised status? Then again, the immunocompromised status that made them more susceptible could be related to age, their cancer, or, in this case, probably both. Could it also be due to the person not having the antibodies for the virus due to not receiving the flu vaccine? Also, even if he or she did receive the vaccine, would it have been effective considering vaccines often work better on healthier, less immunocompromised individuals? Was it due to the more sedentary lifestyle in a nursing care facility that fails to promote healthier lifestyles that may enhance immunity? We can continue, but this should be enough to demonstrate the difficulty in finding cause. Real-life situations are not like a controlled experiment that can isolate the extraneous variables involved. Thus, often we have to speak of causes or associative or correlational findings that do not allow us to say, definitively, "this single element A leads to B." When we attempt to understand and find the cause of an infection, we have to use the Humian definition of cause, put forth by David Hume, as cause being a "constant conjunction" between two or more events.

In science, the way that one finds cause is through a controlled experiment, but infectious agents and people acquiring these agents in healthcare settings are far removed from nice, clean, controlled experimental conditions. Nevertheless, science, including scientific investigation of infection and microbial agents, frequently employs three major types of causes: sufficient cause, necessary cause, and necessary and sufficient cause.

A sufficient cause states that for B to occur, A must occur. A is therefore necessary for B. If A (the heart is diseased) then B (there will be inadequate tissue oxygenation in the body). If the heart cannot pump adequately to maintain the circulatory demands of the blood to pump oxygenated blood to areas of the body, this will lead to inadequate oxygenation, and the person will become hypoxic. However, A is sufficient to explain B, but because B could have occurred in other ways, A was not necessary. For instance, moving to very high altitudes will lead to reduction in oxygenation. COPD can lead to reduced oxygenation. Carbon dioxide or carbon monoxide inhalation will lead to reduced perfusion of oxygen within the tissues. There are many more things that can lead to the consequence of reduced or lack of tissue oxygenation or individuals being hypoxic.

Now, this explanation of sufficient cause leads to even greater complexity. There is often a large set of conditions that are involved in the cause. Furthermore, a single cause can lead to a large number of consequences or effects. Let us examine the set of conditions related to cause first.

I turn on my car and it starts. Without the keys I could not start the car. But are the keys the only causative factor involved in the consequence of starting the car? The keys are involved in initiating, or tripping the spark that leads to the plugs firing, which are also dependent on the electrical integrity of the plug wires being intact. Even if all of this is in place, what if the car did not have a battery? Also, if there is no gas, the car is not going to turn over and go anywhere. And what if all of these things are working properly and your fuel line is blocked? All of these things, as well as many more, have to be in place for the final effect, the car starting. Therefore, cause is often predicated not just on any one element, but many elements. The same applies to infection and infection control. Subsequently, in reality, cause is often not just a single variable, but a set of conditions. This can be demonstrated as follows:

A (A1, A2, A3, A4, A5, . . .), then B

In the above, (A) is the cause in totality. Notice that the cause in totality is made up of many elements that in their own right are causative as well.

When we speak of cause, we also speak of an effect as well. Here again there is considerable complexity. Often, no single cause leads to just one singular effect, and a single cause does not just have a single outcome, but outcomes. Think about getting a promotion that allows you to earn $50,000 more a year. That $50,000 now leads to you moving your children from public to private schools. It leads to you buying a new house. You place a down payment on a new car. You are able to see your physician and dentist for preventative services that you were formerly not able to have. Your family can now take that vacation you have wanted to go on for a few years. More things could be added to this example, but suffice it to say, the antecedent or cause (the $50,000 annual raise) led to a whole array of consequences.

A (the cause) leads to B (B1, B2, B3, B4, B5, . . .)

Notice that a single event causes an array of effects. B, the totality of the effect that was caused by A is not really a single entity, but the effect is made up of an array of elements. In infection control parlance, think about a microbial infection leading to a febrile state, an inflammation, a person being septic, the resident experiencing shock, and cardiovascular insufficiency, just to mention a few.

Now are you starting to see the complexity of cause? These are things that infection control specialists have to be aware of in examining situations. Our reductionist thinking makes us always want to conceptualize a single cause leading to a single effect. Life would be so easy if things always worked on that premise. However, this is far more the exception then the rule.

Now let us take a look at another causal precept: Cause as necessary. Previously we spoke of cause as a sufficient condition. Now, as a necessary condition we can view cause as such: If B, then A, however, if not A, then not B. For example, if you have the H1N1 type of influenza, then you have the virus for H1N1 influenza strain. However, if you do not have the H1N1 influenza virus, you cannot have the H1N1 type of influenza.

Even with the necessary condition for cause, there is a level of complexity that has to be acknowledged. If the person has influenza and it is found to be the H1N1 strain, then the person has the H1N1 virus for this type of influenza. If the person has influenza and no H1N1 virus is found, then the person does not have the H1N1 virus, but he or she may have another strain of influenza. Furthermore, everyone who has the H1N1 strain of influenza has the H1N1 virus. However, many individuals harbor the H1N1 virus but viral symptoms are never manifest in these individuals. Therefore, the condition for getting H1N1 is necessary, but it is not necessary and sufficient. Often there needs to be more involved than just harboring that strain of virus.

Now the strictest test of cause is often referred to as meeting the standards of both being necessary and sufficient. This can be defined as such: If A, then B, and if not A, then not B. Whenever A occurs, B will occur, and if A does not occur, B cannot happen. Most individuals, in doing causal analysis, including infection control causal analysis, think on this level. In reality, the necessary and sufficient cause is often more commonly found in laboratory conditions. Attempting to find such a condition within healthcare institutions as it applies to cause of infections is far more fleeting. There are so many confounding factors that can influence causal analysis that finding a necessary and sufficient condition is far from a reality in this area. It does not mean that it cannot happen. However, in most cases, the factors leading to results are based on multiple causes and multiple effects.

Other facets of cause

Let me examine a few other facets of cause. Many things that are thought to be the cause may not be the cause at all. We have already mentioned that attempting to find a single cause is often quite elusive. Many times the best we can do is to determine a correlation, an association between two or more variables, which is not technically a cause. Correlation does not mean causation. It just means that two or more variables are related, such as height and weight. It does not tell us if A caused B or B caused A, or if a third variable affected the relationship. However, many correlating factors may be contributing factors to a larger cause. Here again, attempting to extrapolate a single cause and effect is more fallacious than realistic. Suppose a person tests positive for beta strep, and has strep throat. The bacteria caused this, correct? Well, not so fast. Many people can harbor the bacteria and never get ill. So now we look at this person who has strep throat. We see he was working 70 hours each week. He was only getting three to four hours of sleep each night. He was often having a diet of fast food with little fruit and vegetables and high levels of fat content. He also going through a divorce, which led to increased levels of stress. Here again, what is the definitive cause? What if he was treated with an antibiotic and the microorganism is eradicated, only to come back two weeks later and cause another infection? Is it now due to the microorganism, to all the other unremitting features that have not abated, or a combination of both? Strep throat is caused by the streptococcal bacteria, but in this case, would the person have even have had the first infection if he did not have all the other contributing factors?

Another type of cause to examine is proximal cause. Attorneys often like to use proximal cause in determining criminal cause or negligence. Proximal means "close to." We often will jump at things that are closely associated in time and even distance to a particular state. For example, a person gets a vaccine and, a few hours later, feels ill and runs a fever. Many people will say they received the influenza vaccine and subsequently got the flu. With the current influenza vaccines, this is not usually going to be the case, but the proximal relationship of the vaccine to feeling sick often makes individuals jump to claim cause. A proximal cause may exist, which may lead to an infection. However, the proximal cause is just the final sequence of factors that have led in a contributory fashion to the illness. In the case of the person experiencing flu-like symptoms after receiving the vaccine, the vaccine was not the cause, but possibly it is manufactured by a psychosomatic state and expectancy of the individual that they were going to get the flu when they received the vaccine, or perhaps they were already getting the flu prior to obtaining the vaccine, or there are a whole host of other things that can explain this situation.

Some Common Techniques to Help Quantify Your Analysis

Many individuals who gather data for any QA/QI purpose fail to properly understand how to bring the data together and how to interpret the findings. Subsequently, many forms of QI data suffer from the old adage, "junk in, junk out." As our discussion of cause demonstrated, data analysis, which so-called causal analysis is part of, cannot be taken haphazardly. It must be well-organized, structured, clear, and reflect what is under examination. All too often, baseless conclusions are drawn. In this final section of the book, I would like to provide a brief examination of data analysis and provide some very basic, yet highly useful, techniques for data analysis as it relates to infection control.

First, confusion often exists between what data is and what data shows. Data is just what exists—the bare facts. For instance, if a gram stain came back indicating that the bacteria cultured was a "gram negative" microbe, this is a fact. This is what was revealed by the procedure.

Data is the facts that were found. However, many individuals misinterpret a "fact" with a "truth." Facts and truths are two different things. Just because something was found to be a fact does not mean it is indicative of the truth. In the above example, a person has a culture that revealed a "gram negative" bacterium. That is a fact. However, suppose the person was demonstrating paralysis with clinical features of poliomyelitis, and, upon further testing, they isolated the polio viral agent responsible for the paralysis and confirmed poliomyelitis. It was a fact that the person did have a gram stain indicating a gram negative organism. That fact is the truth only in relation to the gram negative organism. The truth of the malady as it existed in the person was due to signs and symptoms that were more consistent with what the reality of the illness was—poliomyelitis. The confirmation of this diagnosis was further enhanced by isolating the viral agent responsible for poliomyelitis—a fact. Facts hold a unit of information, but nothing more. It is up to the person examining the data, whether it is a physician, a laboratory technician, a researcher, or an infection control specialist, to take a number of facts and fit and connect them to each other in order to make sense of the information and ascertain the truth as it relates to the reality that one is examining.

Another common error is made when individuals state that the data are, in themselves, telling us something. This is often reflected by statements such as "the data show," "what the data are telling us," and "the data speaks for itself," as well as "the data confirm." These statements invoke data with a power that it, by itself, does not have. Furthermore, many will say "the data are the facts; you can't dispute facts." Well, yes you can. Because a fact, as we mentioned above, is just something that is—and by itself it does not reflect whether it is a piece of data that was obtained without mistake or bias, or even whether the fact or data is connected to what one is looking to explain.

Data does not speak. Data by itself does not show. Data by itself does not confirm. It is up to the person who is investigating (in this case, investigating infection control issues) to take the data, organize them, and determine whether they reflect a particular reality. It is the person who takes the data and makes sense of it. It is the person who takes the data and uses it to understand the truth. When a resident is demonstrating signs and symptoms of tuberculosis and a sputum sample is completed with an acid-fast procedure that comes back positive for the acid-fast tuberculosis bacterium, then the clinical signs, the patient symptoms, and the clinical laboratory specimen test results—all individuals facts that are found to exist—must be organized by a physician, lab technician, researcher, etc., to provide a diagnosis, a level of truth, about why the resident is so ill.

Hopefully this brief discussion helps to illuminate the importance of understanding what data is, what a fact is, and the role a person such as an infection control coordinator has in adequately understanding these areas, as well as the role he or she plays in taking this information, organizing it, and providing an explanation.

Given the previous information, we can now provide some information about data analysis. Here again, this is a very expansive area that cannot be covered in great detail in this book. Yet, this author would like to convey some basic understanding of data analysis and provide briefly some tools that can be used to help with the data analysis.

I would like to start with a big misconception that is often found, not just in infection control, but in all areas of research. Individuals have a tendency to attempt to use the most complex procedures and explanations when other much more simple procedures will work just as well, if not better. We should be guided by William of Occam and the law referred to as "Occam's razor." This states that often the most simple, straightforward method and explanation is the best. Too often, individuals think that using sophisticated techniques, many of which may be used quite inappropriately, will in some way provide greater credence to their results. This is wrong and this type of thinking should be checked and corrected. However, this does not mean that everything needs to be made as simple as possible. For sure, some things are not amenable to base simplicity. Occam's razor states that we should not make issues more complex, or use procedures that are unnecessarily "excessively" complex, when a clearer, much simpler procedure will do the job.

This book does not lend itself to delineating the large array of data analysis tools that can be utilized for infection control investigation. I am only going to introduce some basic, but nevertheless important, statistical procedures that can be used to help an infection control specialist in long-term care. Remember the admonition above, just because they are basic does not mean they are less useful than more sophisticated procedures.

When conducting an infection control investigation, one should attempt to place the data into a measurable, quantifiable realm. Data that lends itself to quantification is subsequently able to lend itself to greater precision in measurement. Our ability to numerically quantify the data and place it in a mathematical form, so that it can be measured, is the cornerstone of scientific research. However, neither the data, nor the statistical or measuring tool, can supplant the knowledge of the person who is doing the investigation and who ultimately has to make sense of the data and the measurements that have been taken. Keep this in mind. Remember that the person in charge of overseeing infection control and investigation infection control issues is ultimately the person who controls the process and makes sense of any analyses that is done.

Some Simple Statistical Procedures to Help With Infection Control Analysis

Let us now take a look at some simple quantitative tools that, although not highly sophisticated, can provide some very nice and insightful feedback on examining infection control issues within your healthcare facility. The purpose here is to enhance the quantitative ability for those engaged in the practice of QA/QI and infection control by providing some clear and simple tools that can be readily understood. Let us take a look at the first tool, the bar graph.

Bar graph

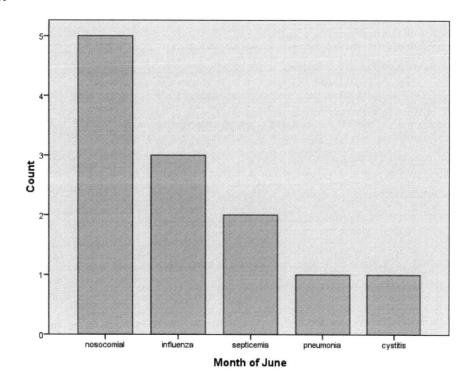

The above is a bar graph. It is a simple tool. On the horizontal axis, or X axis, is the independent variable, and on the vertical axis, or Y axis, is the dependent variable. The independent variable, causes or is instrumental in leading to the effect; the dependent variable is found on the vertical, or Y axis. In this case we are looking at the number (which is often referred to as nominal scale data since it is a total count of each element) of specific types of infections. I simplified it and used only five types of infections. For the month of June, there were five cases of nosocomial infections, three cases of influenza, two cases of septicemia, and one case each of pneumonia and cystitis.

Remember, the above, has been simplified for this example. In reality, there will likely be many more cases of infection in a given month, especially based on the size, age, and acuity of the population. However, the bar graph provides a nice illustration of the type and number of infections in the facility. Visualizing the data helps in its examination. Note, this is a descriptive statistical technique that just describes what was found to exist in the facility in a given month. What would be needed further is an examination of other months and the number and types of infections that existed to see if this month's (June) number demonstrated any appreciable change and why.

Line graph

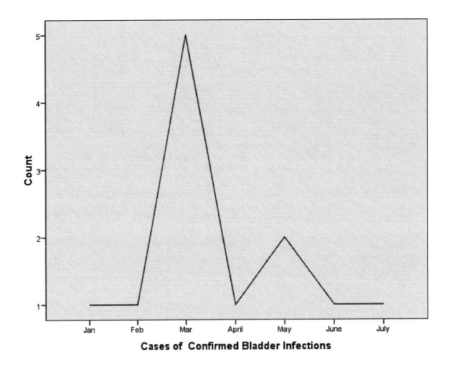

Cases of Confirmed Bladder Infections

The above line graph is another simple descriptive tool. The line graph is examining the trend of confirmed bladder infections for the first seven months of a particular year. It is a good tool to use to illustrate trends when examining one particular infection control issue. The horizontal axis, or X axis, shows the month, and the vertical axis, or Y axis, shows the count of the total number of infections for each month. As one can see, there were two spikes, and othe spike in March was considerable. There are several questions that could be asked based on the line graph's data. For instance, does the data demonstrate a level of control on this issue (bladder infections)? Is it markedly different from other periods that have been examined and, if so, how (i.e., better, worse, or no major changes)? Was March's spike due to a reason that could be isolated? These are just some of the questions that can be raised when examining this line graph.

Scatter plot and correlation

As I mentioned, often it is difficult, if not impossible, to find a definitive cause. In many cases, the best we can find is a correlation, or a relationship between two or more variables. Although correlation is not causation, it can still provide valuable information. All correlations are measured on a scale ranging from negative 1.0 to positive 1.0. The closer to negative or positive 1.0, the stronger the correlation. A zero reading indicates no correlation. Providing a visual display of the data being examined to see if any relationship exists. Let me provide this scenario: Suppose that you wanted to examine the relationship between the number of infections found in your facility for a given month as it relates to the monthly hours per patient day, or PPD, a common method used to calculated hours staffing to resident. The infection control coordinator has the average PPDs for each month in a particular year; she also has the number of infections that were found in the facility each month for that given year. Here is the data:

Month	PPD	Number of Infections
January	2.90	25.00
February	3.50	21.00
March	3.60	22.00
April	3.10	26.00
May	2.80	32.00
June	2.95	29.00
July	3.20	23.00
August	3.50	28.00
September	3.70	20.00
October	2.99	29.00
November	2.80	28.00
December	3.20	24.00

Given this information, you can create a scatter plot. PPDs will be placed on the horizontal axis, or X axis, and number of infections will be placed on the vertical axis, or Y axis. When completed, you will have the following results:

Month infection rate to HPPD

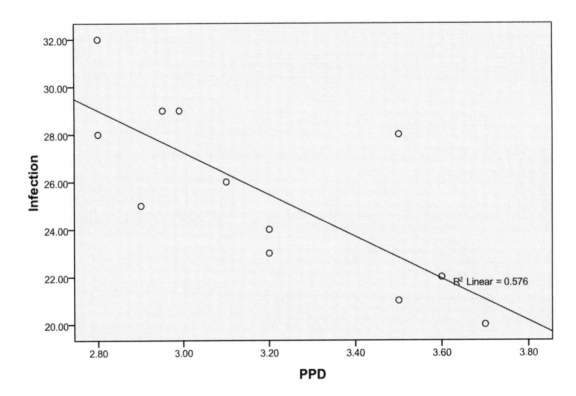

Looking at the results, it's clear that a correlation exists. If no or very little correlation existed, the data would not have any direction, and would almost take on a circular look. However, in this case, you can see that the data are leaning toward the left. What this means is that low scores on the X axis are related, generally speaking, to greater amounts of infections found as evident on the Y axis. This shows a strong negative relation. In this case, what the information shows is when the two types of data are plotted in association to each other, what is found to exist, generally speaking, is that as PPDs go down, or fewer hours of care are given to each resident, the number of infections for a given month tended to increase.

Negative relationship just means that, generally speaking, as data on the X axis become smaller, data on the Y axis becomes larger, and vice versa. This is sometimes referred to as an inverse relationship. This is in contrast to a positive or direct relationship where if X goes up, Y does as well, and as X goes down, Y does too. When one hears positive or negative, one should not think of something being better or worse or imputing some type of value statement. All negative or positive relationships mean is whether it is an inverse or direct relationship between the two variables.

As mentioned previously, all correlations range from a negative 1.0 to positive 1.0. Negative 1.0 indicates a perfect, but inverse relationship between two variables. A positive 1.0 correlation indications a perfect and direct relationship between two variables. This indicates that each movement of data on X is matched by an opposite direction of movement found on Y. Conversely, a positive 1.0 is a perfect positive relationship, which indicates that for each movement of data on X, the corresponding data of Y move in the same direction. In reality, perfect correlations are almost never seen.

You may have noticed the line that is going through the data. This is referred to as a regression line. It acts like a floating mean, which provides a visual average of the slope of the line based on the data, and it is the line of best fit that minimized the distance around the line, which is the line of best fit that minimizes the distance of the data points that the line intersects through. The line is calculated based on its mathematical slope. Notice also the line, as many of you may have learned from algebra, is moving from high on the left to a lower level as it moves to the right. This further shows the negative correlation found in the data.

The correlation of the above data can also be mathematically quantified. It is not a difficult procedure, but it can be tedious if you have a large amount of information. However, programs such as Excel or other statistics programs can do the calculations, as well as the scatter plot, quite quickly after data is entered. Below are the mathematical results of the data that are reflected in the above scatter plot.

Correlations			PPD	Infection
PPD	Pearson Correlation		1	-.759**
	Sig. (2-tailed)			.004
	N		12	12
Infection	Pearson Correlation		-.759**	1
	Sig. (2-tailed)		.004	
	N		12	12

** Correlation is significant at the 0.01 level (2-tailed).

For those who like a "hard number," this data analysis provides it. We could see that the correlation in the scatter plot was strong, but just how strong was it? Without a mathematical calculation, this was hard to precisely determine. However, we can see that the correlation between PPDs and infection was a negative 0.759, which is a very strong relationship. This means that, generally speaking, X was inversely related to Y, or that as PPDs became smaller, infections increased and vice versa.

Finding averages

Finding averages is a very simple, yet highly important, procedure. It helps to provide a benchmark of where you are currently, and allows you to compare what your current (average) results are in relation to other months, years, or to other healthcare organizations in your state or country. The common ways to look at averages are the mean, median, and mode. They are often referred to as measures of central tendency because they show where your central, or average, scores fall.

The mean

The mean is what most people think of when they think of an average. It is sometimes called the arithmetic mean. It is defined as the sum of a set of scores divided by the total number of observations. For instance, say you want to determine the average number of infections that are found in a given year. Suppose the following were the total infections found in your facility each month:

January	=	20
February	=	30
March	=	15
April	=	20
May	=	25
June	=	30
July	=	10
August	=	12
September	=	18
October	=	20
November	=	25
December	=	30

The following formula represents the mean: bar X equals the summation of X/N.

If you add all the months for the entire year, the total is 255. When you divide 255 by 12 months you have a mean of 21.25. Therefore, your healthcare facility for the given year averaged 21.25 infections each month. You have just created a nice average. How does that average compare to other facilities of similar size and with a similar patient acuity level? How do you compare on a county, state, or national level?

The median

The median is also very easy to figure out. It is the score that is at the middlemost part of a distribution of scores—that is, 50% of the scores fall above the median and 50% fall below. For instance, using the preceding example you would find the median by first ranking the scores from highest to lowest—30, 30, 30, 25, 25, 20, 20, 20, 18, 15, 12, 10. Given these scores, the median is found by looking at the distribution. There are 12 numbers. Therefore, you count six down or six up. Six numbers down and six up are 20 and 20. You would add those two numbers and divide by two and the median is 20. If the distribution of numbers was an odd distribution, for instance 11 numbers, you would go five down and five up and the number in between those two numbers would be the median.

The median is less likely to be inflated by a couple of extreme values. For instance, if you had a set of scores such as 10, 20, 20, 30, 150, the median would be 20, but the mean would be 46 since the 150, the extreme score, inflated the average. Since the mean is more sensitive to extreme variations, one or two extreme scores could artificially inflate the average.

The mode

The mode is the score that appears most frequently in a given distribution. In looking at the 12 months of documented infections, we can again see the following monthly counts:

January	=	20
February	=	30
March	=	15
April	=	20
May	=	25
June	=	30
July	=	10
August	=	12
September	=	18
October	=	20
November	=	25
December	=	30

There are three months that had 30 infections, two months that had 25 infections, three months that had 20 infections, one month that had 18 infections, one month that had 15 infections, one month that had 12 infections, and one month that had 10 infections. There are actually two sets of numbers that come up at the highest frequency. There are three months during which 30 infections were found and three months during which 20 infections were found. Therefore, there are actually two modes, 20 and 30.

Comparative analysis in isolating cause

John Stuart Mill, the prominent utilitarian philosopher, developed a system of logic that is still used today. He developed two major methods for making logical comparisons, which he referred to as the method of agreement and the method of difference. These approaches seek to give a causal explanation by examining the regularities within the particular context under examination (Neuman, 2000). Through examining points of agreement and differences, individuals are able to help isolate causal patterns or particular cases. I will examine both of these methods separately for the reader.

The method of agreement

In using the method of agreement to examine infection control, the infection control personnel investigating a particular issue will focus their attention on what is common across a number of cases. In the example given here, let us say that the infection control committee is concerned about why there has been such a high rate of cystitis over the past few months. In examining this issue, they undertake a comparative analysis. When doing comparative analysis, you look at each case in which a person was diagnosed with cystitis. You examine a number of variables, such as hydration levels, diagnosis, catheter use, medications, staff training, etc. Each of the letters in the following table stands for a particular variable that is coded and represented by the letter. For instance, if the person had a catheter, maybe we would code that with an (a), poor hydration (b), and so on.

You would often have a number of cases that would be under investigation. For our purpose, I have just used four. Each case represents a resident who had a diagnosed case of cystitis. As I have already mentioned, the letters that I used stand for variables, though here I did not specifically define each coded letter. For our purpose using letters will help illustrate how this technique works. However, in reality, you often would use letters, or even numbers, that represent some type of notation for a variable as a shorthand way to analyze the data. Below is the comparative analysis undertaken for cystitis using the method of agreement.

Case 1	Case 2	Case 3	Case 4
a	a	a	a
b	b	b	b
c	c	d	e
f	f	g	h
i	j	k	k
l	m	l	n
o	o	p	q

In the four cases shown here, all four cases of cystitis shared (a) and (b). Let us say that (a) stood for an in-dwelling catheter and (b) dehydration. In looking at the other variables there was considerable variation, but on these two, they were consistently shown to be associated with cases of cystitis found in this long-term care facility. What we may be able to ascertain by this is that the higher rates of cystitis witnessed over the last few months in the long-term care facility are related to (1) indwelling catheters and (2) dehydration. Although we cannot say for sure whether these are the exclusive or only two reasons, we can be fairly confident that there does appear to be a pattern demonstrating a fairly sound logic to view these two reasons as instrumental in the increased rates of cystitis.

The method of difference

In some instances, cases may be in agreement in certain areas and it is not what they share, but what they do not share, that is the most informative. For instance, what happens when we are examining an infectious issue and in looking at the cases, they share great similarity on numerous variables. In such cases, it may behoove the investigator to undertake a method of difference and examine differences, glaring or very subtle, that are not caught by the method of agreement.

The method of difference gives the researcher a stronger ability to understand the logic of causal analysis. It is more or less a "double application" of the method of agreement, in which you first examine cases that share a similarity in many areas, while at the same time being attentive to the differences that are found in crucial areas (Neuman, 2000). By examining those cases that share many features and do not end up with the same results, while paying close attention to some of the subtle discrepancies that may have caused these differences to transpire, you can logically extrapolate, with greater certainty than in the method of agreement, the causal analysis for a particular phenomenon.

Let us say we are examining cases in which individuals either did or did not have a confirmed case of influenza. Using a simple example below, we are looking at four residents. Case 1, case 2, and case 4 all were free of any influenza. However, case 3 did experience a confirmed case of influenza. In examining the variables that affected all four cases, the one difference found in case 3 that was not in case 1, 2, or 4 was that case 3 in row 3 had a coded (d) instead of a coded (c). The (d) in this case meant that resident or case 3 did not receive the influenza vaccine, while cases 1, 2, and 4 did.

Case 1	Case 2	Case 3	Case 4
a	a	a	a
b	b	b	b
c	c	d	c
f	f	f	f
i	i	i	i
l	l	l	l
0	0	0	0

The method of difference is slightly more complicated than the method of agreement, but it offers more powerful logic in causal analysis. We first look at the similarities among the cases, but we closely scrutinize any particular difference that may lead to the results. It is quite similar to saying person A, B, and C went to a restaurant, and A and C had food poisoning. What caused it? If they all ate corn, had a cream source on their vegetables, ate an appetizer of shrimp, had lemon pie, but A and C had salmon and B had steak, they all shared similarity on every-thing they ate except the steak and the salmon. Those who ate the salmon experienced food poisoning and the person who had steak did not. The method of difference is following the same logic only usually in greater detail and often with more variables.

This was a very brief introduction into some techniques that can be employed by infection control personnel to analyze important infection control issues. The statistical procedures that I introduced here are rudimentary, but they may be helpful to many who are attempting to analyze data. However, individuals who are going to be heavily involved in infection control would be well served to enhance their skills in data analysis and become more skilled and conversant with the important, and even more advanced, techniques that will ultimately benefit infection control personnel to become more effective in their positions.

Chapter 8

Resources and References

Introduction

This chapter contains additional information and resources to enhance your agency's program, including the following items:

- A glossary of key terms
- Resources
- References

Glossary

Active immunity

A person's bodily response to an antigen, in which it produces antibodies to a specific antigen. Often confers much longer lasting immunity that passive immunity.

Acute

Diseases or conditions that have a quick onset.

Acquired/adaptive immunity

The immunity achieved through B and T cells, often derived from and differentiated in the lymphoid tissue.

Advisory Committee on Immunization Practices (ACIP)

A committee of the Centers for Disease Control and Prevention that issues immunization guidelines and recommendations, including indications for vaccinations, administration protocols, precautions, and contraindications.

Aerosolized

Spread through the air.

Agent

The source or cause of a disease or infection.

AIDS

Acquired immunodeficiency syndrome.

Amniotic fluid

The fluid that surrounds the fetus throughout pregnancy.

Antibody

An immunoglobulin produced by lymphocytes in response to bacteria, viruses, or other antigenic substances.

Asepsis

The absence of germs; the removal or destruction of disease-producing organisms or infected material.

Bacteria

Any of the small, unicellular microorganisms of the class Schizomycetes.

Bag technique

Principles for handling a nursing/staff bag that prevent contamination.

B-cells

Cells of the acquired or adaptive immune system derived from the bone marrow and often become plasma cells

Betadine®

A trademark for the topical anti-infective providone-iodine.

Blood

Any human blood, blood components, or products made from blood.

Bloodborne pathogens

Infectious microorganisms that can cause disease in humans. They can be present in blood, blood products, semen, cerebrospinal fluid, synovial fluid, pericardial fluid, amniotic fluid, vaginal drainage, and other body fluids that are visibly contaminated with blood, such as urine, stool, emesis, saliva, sputum, and wound drainage. Transmission occurs through contact with contaminated blood or body fluids in the healthcare setting by needlesticks, through breaks in the skin, or from splashes into the mouth, nose, or eyes. Transmission also occurs through needle sharing, through sexual contact, and from mother to fetus during pregnancy. Viruses spread by bloodborne pathogens include hepatitis B, hepatitis C, and human immunodeficiency virus.

Body fluids

Fluids from the human body (other than blood). Includes emesis, sputum, feces, urine, semen, vaginal secretions, nasal secretions, saliva, sweat, tears, cerebrospinal fluid, synovial fluid, pleural fluid, pericardial fluid, amniotic fluid, and breast milk.

Body substance isolation

A component of standard precautions that reduces the risk of transmitting pathogens from moist body substances.

Cardiopulmonary resuscitation (CPR)

A basic emergency procedure for life support, consisting of artificial respiration and manual external cardiac massage.

Carrier

A person that harbors the disease, but may not present any signs or symptoms of the microbial/infectious agent.

Cell-mediated immunity

Immunity that is often produced through T-cell cytotoxity, through cell-to-cell contact.

Centers for Disease Control and Prevention (CDC)

A federal agency of the U.S. government that provides facilities and services for the investigation, identification, prevention, and control of disease.

Cerebrospinal fluid

Fluid that flows through and protects the brain and spinal canal.

Chronic

Conditions or diseases that often come on slower than acute diseases and stay for longer durations of time.

Communicable diseases

Diseases that are transferrable between individuals.

Contaminated laundry

Laundry that is soiled with blood or other potentially infectious materials, or that may contain sharps.

Contamination

A condition of being soiled, stained, touched, or otherwise exposed to harmful agents, such as bloodborne pathogens.

Crackles

Common, abnormal respiratory sound heard on auscultation of the chest during inspiration.

Decontamination

The use of physical or chemical means to remove, inactivate, or destroy bloodborne pathogens on a surface/item so that it is no longer capable of transmitting infectious particles; the surface or item then is rendered safe for handling, use, or disposal.

Direct transmission

Exposure to a microbial agent without any mediating influence. This is typically person-to-person contact.

Disinfect

To remove pathogens.

Disinfectant

A chemical applied to objects that destroys microorganisms and removes pathogens.

E. coli

Abbreviation for *Escherichia coli,* a species of coliform bacteria of the family *Enterobacteriaceae,* normally present in the bowels and common in water, milk, and ground.

Employee health

A component of the agency's infection control program, that includes policies and procedures for surveillance, prevention, and control of infection for staff.

Engineering controls

Controls (e.g., sharps disposal containers, self-sheathing needles) that isolate or remove the bloodborne pathogens hazard from the workplace.

Epidemiology

The study of the incidence, demographic arrangement, and causes of disease in humans.

Exposure

Contact with blood or other potentially infectious body fluid that can enter the bloodstream through breaks in the skin, open wounds, mucous membranes, or puncture with an instrument contaminated with blood or body fluids.

Exposure control plan

A written plan that includes a list of high-risk job classifications, tasks, and procedures for evaluating exposure incidents. The agency must review the plan at least once a year, or any time during the year that a procedure changes and affects exposure risk.

Exposure incident

A specific contact with the eye, mouth, other mucous membrane, or non-intact skin, or a parenteral contact with blood or other potentially infectious material that occurs during the performance of an employee's duties.

Flora

Microorganisms that live on or inside the body; they compete with disease-producing microorganisms to provide a natural immunity against some infections.

Fomite

An inanimate object that can hold and transfer infectious agents.

Fungi

A term used to classify organisms requiring an external source of carbon that can invade both humans and nonliving organic substances. They can be single or multi-cell organisms with distinctive cell wall features.

Hand washing

The act of cleansing the hands of microorganisms by washing them with soap and water or an antiseptic solution.

Hazardous waste

Material, such as biological substances, that can transmit disease (infectious waste), radioactive materials, or toxic chemicals; dangerous to humans and other living organisms and requires special precautions for disposal.

HBV

Virus that causes hepatitis B.

HCV

Virus that causes hepatitis C.

Helminths

Parasitic worm infections.

Hepatitis B vaccine

A vaccine designed to help a person develop immunity from HBV. Advised for people likely to come in contact with blood and body fluids.

HIV

Human immunodeficiency virus that causes AIDS.

Host

That which harbors a disease causing agent, such as a person or animal.

Household bleach

All-purpose disinfectant for blood and body fluid spills and decontamination. Dilute one part bleach with 10 parts water.

Humoral immunity

Produced through plasma cells and antibodies attacking antigens.

Iatrogenic infections

Those caused by the healthcare providers themselves, in their interaction with patients/residents.

Indirect transmission

A mediating factor is involved, such as a person leaving microbial agents on a door knob, that when contacted by another person, lead to the person becoming infected.

Immune response

A defense function of the body that produces antibodies to destroy invading antigens and malignancies.

Immunization

A process by which resistance to an infectious disease is induced or augmented.

Immunocompromised

Pertaining to an immune response that has been weakened by a disease or immunosuppressive agent, such as chemotherapy.

Incubation period

The period during which the microorganism is often replicating.

Infection

Invasion of the body by pathogenic microorganisms.

Infection control program

An agency's program, including policies and procedures, for surveillance, prevention, and control of infection for staff, patients, families, and caregivers.

Innate immunity

Immunity that were are born with, often related to our skin as a barrier and the white blood cells that derive from the myeloid tissue.

Latency period

A period of dormancy where the person may not be symptomatic but yet they are still carrying the infectious agent and potentially a vector for infecting others.

Latex

An emulsion or fluid-like sap produced in special cells or vessels of certain plants. Latex contains resins, proteins, and other substances and is a source of rubber.

Memory cells

Part of humoral immunity and the B-cell lineage that provides a memory (anamestic) response to recognize antigenic agents previously encountered.

Microorganisms

Any tiny, microscopic entity capable of carrying on living processes. They can be of pathogenic nature.

Mode of transmission

The vehicle pathogens use to travel from one reservoir to another to spread infection.

Methicillin-resistant staphylococcus aureus (MRSA)

A strain of *Staphylococcus aureus* that is resistant to penicillins, cephalosporins, and most other antibiotics except vancomycin.

Mycobacterium tuberculosis (TB)

A bacillus that causes a disease through airborne droplet nuclei that infect the lungs after being inhaled.

National Institute for Occupational Safety and Health (NIOSH)

Part of the Centers for Disease Control and Prevention; the single federal institute responsible for conducting research and making recommendations for the prevention of work-related illnesses and injuries.

Nosocomial infections

Infections that are acquired by being a patient/resident within a healthcare environment.

Occupational exposure

Reasonably anticipated skin, eye, mucous membrane, or parenteral contact with blood or other potentially infectious materials that may occur during the performance of an employee's duties.

Occupational Safety and Health Administration (OSHA)

Agency of the U.S. Department of Labor responsible for creating and enforcing workplace safety and health regulations.

Opportunistic

Organisms that often will not cause disease in healthy individuals but rely on individuals that have compromised immune responses to cause disease.

Oral barrier

Mechanical emergency respiratory devices designed to isolate a caregiver from contact with potentially infectious substances.

Other potentially infectious material

Any fluid that may potentially contain blood or other body secretions.

Parenteral

Piercing the skin or mucous membranes through such means as needlesticks, cuts or abrasions, or human bites.

Passive immunity

Antibodies from another source transferred to someone to confer, often a shorter, temporary immune response.

Pathogen

Any microorganism capable of producing disease.

Performance improvement

(See Quality improvement.)

Pericardial fluid

The lubricating fluid in the sac that surrounds the heart.

Personal protective equipment (PPE)

Garments, gloves, masks, and eyewear designed to create a barrier between caregiver and patient to prevent the spread of infection by bloodborne pathogens.

Personal respirator

The type of mask required by the Occupational Safety and Health Administration for healthcare workers who provide care for patients with tuberculosis. The mask is fitted for individual use after a special fit-test specific for tuberculosis respirator masks.

Plasma cells

Cells that derive from B-cells that are engaged in humoral immunity

Portal of entry

The point where pathogens enter a new reservoir to spread infection.

Portal of exit

Pathogens' exit route from the reservoir to infect other hosts.

Prevention

A future-oriented strategy that improves quality and performance with the goal of decreasing the probability of diseases or accidents.

    a)   Primary prevention—seeks to prevent any type of disease or infection before it starts
    b)   Secondary prevention—seeks to address and ameliorate the disease and symptomatic process.
    c)   Tertiary prevention—seeks to use palliative features to control and prevent any further exacerbations in the condition.

Prion

The smallest infectious agent that exists that, like a virus, is not a living organism, but unlike a virus, only has a protein and no nucleic acids.

Prophylactic

Measures taken to guard against or prevent disease.

Protozoa

Single-celled microorganisms of the class Protozoa, the lowest form of animal life.

Quality improvement (QI)

The ongoing assessment of processes and outcomes to identify opportunities for improvement and institute actions to improve the quality of care. Also known as performance improvement.

Reservoir

The environment in which pathogens survive. The environment can be a human or animal body, or a medium such as dust.

Rickettsia

A genus of microorganisms that combine aspects of both bacteria and viruses.

Risk management

The process of making and carrying out decisions that will minimize the adverse effects of accidental losses on an organization, and prevent harmful incidents from occurring to workers or customers.

Salmonella

A genus of motile, gram-negative, rod-shaped bacteria, including species that cause typhoid fever and gastroenteritis.

Sharps

Any needles, scalpels, or other objects that could cause wounds or punctures to personnel handling them.

Source individual

A person who may be a source of occupational exposure to workers.

Sputum

Material coughed up from the lungs and expectorated out of the mouth.

Standard precautions

A key component of the Centers for Disease Control and Prevention's guidelines for isolation precautions in hospitals; combines the features of universal precautions and body substance isolation.

Sterile

The absence of all microbes.

Sterilization

Technique for destroying microorganisms using heat, water, chemicals, or gases.

Suctioning

The aspiration of a gas or fluid by reducing air pressure over its surface, usually by mechanical means.

Surveillance

The ongoing monitoring of infections to detect changes in trends or distribution in order to initiate investigations or control measures for noted variances.

Susceptible host

A predisposition or sensitivity to the effects of infectious diseases, allergens, or other pathogenic agents; lacking adequate immunity or resistance. Individuals fitting this description require close observation or examination.

Synovial fluid

The lubricating fluid of joints, bursae, and tendon sheaths.

T-cells

A type of lymphoid lineage cell that has many different purposes for immunity. The two most commonly mentioned are T-helper (CD4) and T-cytotoxic (CD8).

Titer

The strength of a solution or substance established through titration.

Tracking and trending

A process by which to measure the effectiveness of the infection control program.

Tuberculosis (TB)

A chronic infection caused by the mycobacterium tuberculosis usually affecting the lungs and generally transmitted by inhalation of infected droplets.

Typhus

Any of a group of acute infectious diseases caused by various species of Rickettsia and usually transmitted from infected rodents to humans by the bites of lice, fleas, mites, or ticks.

Universal precautions

An approach to infection control designed to prevent transmission of bloodborne diseases, initially developed in 1987 by the Centers for Disease Control and Prevention. This approach describes protective work practices that should be followed by anyone who comes into contact with a patient. These practices treat all human blood and certain body fluids as if they are known to be infectious for HIV, HBV, HCV, and/or other bloodborne pathogens.

Urinary meatus

The external opening of the urethra.

Vancomycin-resistant Enterococcus (VRE)

A strain of *Enterococcus* which is resistant to most antibiotics, including vancomycin.

Vector

A carrier, especially one that transmits disease.

Vehicles

Nonliving objects that are instrumental in the transfer of disease-causing agents.

Virulence

The potency of a disease causing agent.

Virus

A very small, yet very complex, parasitic nonliving agent, made up of DNA or RNA and a protein coat that has no independent metabolic activity; it can replicate only within a cell of a living plant or animal host.

Work practice controls

Controls that reduce the likelihood of exposure by altering the manner in which a task is performed (e.g., prohibiting the recapping of needles by using a two-handed technique).

Zoonosis

An animal agent that harbors and infectious agent and transfers it to a human, usually used to refer to a transfer of an microbial agent from a vertebrate animal to a human.

Resources

American College of Allergy, Asthma and Immunology

http://acaai.org/

An educational resource for every aspect of allergy, asthma, and immunology treatment, and an excellent source for latex sensitivity information

American Lung Association

800-LUNGUSA

http://www.lung.org/

Health agency that provides education, advocacy, and research on TB and other respiratory diseases

Association for Professionals in Infection Control and Epidemiology, Inc.

http://www.apic.org/

A multidisciplinary international organization dedicated to prevention of infectious diseases through education, research, practice, and credentialing

Centers for Disease Control and Prevention

Hepatitis branch:

http://www.cdc.gov/hepatitis/index.htm

The lead federal agency for protecting public health and safety, offering information on disease control and prevention

Hopkins Medical Products

5 Greenwood Place, Baltimore, MD 21208

800-835-1995

www.hmponline.com

Free catalog that includes disposable gowns and gloves, goggles, resuscitation aids, sharps disposal units, and liquid antiseptic and waterless soaps

National Aids Information Hotline

The hotline can provide information and references for those who would like to learn more about the disease. It is not limited to just those with HIV/AIDS.

National Foundation for Infectious Diseases

301-656-0003

www.nfid.org

A nonprofit organization providing research and support for the cure and prevention of infectious diseases; sponsors public and professional education programs

National Institute of Allergy and Infectious Diseases

www.niaid.nih.gov

An organization of the National Institutes of Health that provides scientists with support in their research on infectious diseases.

Occupational Safety and Health Administration
www.osha.gov
An agency of the U.S. Department of Labor that provides standards and data on health and safety in the workplace environment.

You should also consider your local and county public health departments, your own facility policy and procedure books, as well as you local chapter of the Red Cross as valuable resources for your infection control program.

References

Accreditation Commission for Home Care, Inc. *Multi-Service Accreditation Resource Manual.* Raleigh, NC: ACHC, 1995.

Anderson, Lois E. *Mosby's Medical, Nursing, and Allied Health Dictionary.* 4th ed. St. Louis, MO: Mosby Year Book, Inc., 1994.

Bader, M. S. & McKinsey, D. S. (2005). "Viral infections in the elderly: The challenges of managing herpes zoster, influenza, and RSV." *Postgraduate Medicine* 118, no. 5 (2005).

Beacon Health Corporation. *Homecare Policy Manual for Certification and Accreditation.* Mequon, WI: Beacon Health Corporation, 1997.

————. *Infection Control: Instructor's Guide.* Mequon, WI: Beacon Health Corporation, 1990.

————. *Focus on Infection Control: Instructor's Guide.* Mequon, WI: Beacon Health Corporation, 1992.

————. *Bloodborne Pathogens: Protecting Yourself and Others in Homecare: Instructor's Guide.*

Bauman, Robert W. Microbiology with diseases by body systems. Benjamin Cummings, Boston, MA, 2014.

Mequon, WI: Beacon Health Corporation, 1998.

————. *Homecare Administrative HORIZONS*, vol. 4, nos. 5, 6, 7. Mequon, WI: Beacon Health Corporation, 1997.

————. "Personal Respirators: Policies and Education Improve Compliance." In *Expanded HORIZONS.* Mequon, WI: Beacon Health Corporation, 1995.

Bennett, Gail. "Developing an Effective Infection Control Program for Home Care." *Caring Magazine,* (November 1994): 50–53.

Bowle, Kathy, and Mary Lynch. "These Products and Procedures Prevent Needlesticks." *RN Magazine* (July 1992): 42–45.

Carr, S., Unwin, N. & Pless-Mulloli, T. An introduction to public health and epidemiology. Open University Press, Berkshire, England, 2007.

Centers for Disease Control and Prevention. Hepatitis Surveillance 1978, Rep. 42, 34–36.

———— "Draft Guideline for Infection Control in Healthcare Personnel." *Federal Register* (September 8,1997): 47275–47327.

Centers for Disease Control (CDC) (nd). History of Vaccine Safety. *http://www.cdc.gov/vaccinesafety/Vaccine_Monitoring/history.html*

Centers for Disease Control and Prevention, "Biggest Threats," (n.d.), *http://www.cdc.gov/drugresistance/biggest_threats.html.*

———, "Checklist for Core Elements of Hospital Antibiotic Stewardship Programs," (n.d.), *http://www.cdc.gov/getsmart/healthcare/implementation/checklist.html.*

———, "Core Elements of Hospital Antibiotic Stewardship," (n.d.), *http://www.cdc.gov/getsmart/healthcare/implementation/core-elements.html.*

Centers for Disease Control (CDC). Guideline for infection control in health care personnel, 1998. *http://www.cdc.gov/hicpac/pdf/InfectControl98.pdf.*

Centers for Disease Control. 2016 Recommended Immunizations for Adults: By Age. *http://www.cdc.gov/vaccines/schedules/downloads/adult/adult-schedule-easy-read.pdf.*

Centers for Disease Control. Latex Allergy: A Prevention Guide. *http://www.cdc.gov/niosh/docs/98-113/.*

Centers for Disease Control. CDC - Tuberculosis - NIOSH Workplace Safety and Health. *http://www.cdc.gov/niosh/topics/tb/.*

Charous, B. "The Puzzle of Latex Allergy: Some Answers, Still More Questions." *Annals of Allergy* 73, no. 4: 277–281, 1994.

Community Health Accreditation Program, Inc., and National League for Home Health Care, Inc. *Standards of Excellence for Home Care Organizations.* New York, NY: CHAP, 1993.

Garavaglia, B. The Comprehensive Guide to Nursing Home Administration. HCPro, Danvers, MA, 2012.

Gladwin, Mark, Trattler, William, and Mahan, Scott C. Clinical Microbiology Made Ridiculously Simple (Ed. 6), Miami, FL, 2014.

Goodman, Brenda. *The OSHA Handbook: Interpretive Guidelines for the Bloodborne Pathogen Standard.* El Paso, TX: Skidmore-Roth Publishing, Inc., 1993.

Hanrahan, A., and L. Reutter. "A Critical View of the Literature on Sharps Injuries: Epidemiology, Management of Exposures, and Prevention." *Journal of Advanced Nursing* 25: 144–154, 1997.

Harding, Anne, Pros and Cons of New Hepatitis C Drugs, 2016. *http://www.everydayhealth.com/news/pros-cons-new-hepatitis-treatments-patients/.*

Healthcare Professional Guides: Safety and Infection Control. Springhouse, PA: Springhouse, 1998.

Joint Commission on Accreditation of Healthcare Organizations. *Comprehensive Accreditation Manual for Home Care.* Oakbrook Terrace, IL: JCAHO, 1996.

Keye Productivity Center. *OSHA and the Medical Industry: A Compliance Update.* August 1995.

Knowles, M. S., et al. *Andragogy in Action: Applying Modern Principles of Adult Education.* San Francisco: Jossey-Bass, 1984.

Levinson, Warren. Review of Medical Microbiology and Immunology, Twelfth Edition, Lange Publishing, New York, 2012.

Maki, Dennis G., and George C. Mejicano. "Infections Acquired During Cardiopulmonary Resuscitation: Defining the Risk, Strategies for Prevention." Abstract from the Section of Infectious Diseases, Department of Medicine, University of Wisconsin Medical School University of Wisconsin-Madison, and the Infection Control Department, University of Wisconsin Hospital and Clinics. Madison, WI, 1997.

Medical News Today. Antibiotic resistance in foodborne germs is an ongoing threat, July, 2014. *http://www.medicalnewstoday.com/releases/279112.php.*

Merrill, R. M. (2010). Introduction to epidemiology. Jones and Bartlett Publishers, Sudbury, MA.

Mefford, Jeanette, and Janet Shandeling. *Clinical Procedure Manual for Home Health Agencies.* Minneapolis, MN: Mefford, Knutson & Associates, 1995.

National Institute of Health Education, "Understanding Emerging and Re-emerging Infectious Diseases," (n.d.), *https://science.education.nih.gov/supplements/nih1/diseases/guide/understanding1.html.*

Neuman, William. *Social research methods: qualitative and quantitative approaches.* Boston, Allyn and Bacon, 2000.

Occupational Safety and Health Administration. "Occupational Exposure to Bloodborne Pathogens: Final Rule, 29 CFR, Part 1910, 1030," *Federal Register* (December 6, 1991): 64175–64182.

Occupational Safety and Health Administration (OSHA). Tuberculosis. *https://www.osha.gov/SLTC/tuberculosis/standards.html.*

Omdahl, Diane J. *Headstart to Quality Improvement in Home Care.* Mequon, WI: Beacon Health Corporation, 1997.

Rice, Robyn. *Manual of Home Health Nursing Procedures.* St. Louis, MO: Mosby Year Book, Inc., 1995.

Roop, Joan A. "Implementation of a Hepatitis B Vaccine Program." *Home Health Care Nurse* (July/August 1993).

Roos, R., WHO: Infection control gaps helped fuel UAE MERS surge. Centers for Infectious Disease and Research Policy-CIDRAP, June 2014.

Simmons B, et al. "Infection Control in Home Health Care Settings." *Infection Control and Hospital Epidemiology* 11 (1990): 362–370.

Somerville, M., Kumaran, K. & Anderson, R. Public Health and Epidemiology at a Glance. Wiley-Blackwell. West Sussex, UK, 2012.

Thompson, B. L., et al. "Handwashing and Glove Use in a Long-Term Care Facility." *Infection Control and Hospital Epidemiology* 18 (1997): 97–103.

Thomson Prometric. Certified Professional Food Manager-Course Manual (3rd ed). Thomson Prometric, a part of Thomson Corporation, St. Paul, MN.

Valenti, William M. "Infection Control, HIV and Home Care." *Caring Magazine* (July 1996): 42–47.

Weaver, A. & Goldberg, S. Clincial biostatistics and epidemiology made ridiculously simple. MedMaster, Inc., Miami, Fl, 2012.

World Health Organization (WHO). Practical Guidelines for Infection Control in Healthcare Facilities. *http://www.wpro.who.int/publications/docs/practical_guidelines_infection_control.pdf.*

Wright, J. Williams, R., & Wilkinson, J. R. (1998). Development and importance of health needs assessment. *British Medical Journal,* 316, 1310-1313.